Advance Praise for Diagnosketch

This book is equally as useful to patients as it is to doctors. The illustrations cover the most common diagnoses in the ED and reflect the diversity of patients we see every day. Everyone will find themselves represented here.

—**Thea James, MD, EM Physician; Vice President of Mission and Associate Chief Medical Officer, Boston Medical Center**

Not only does *Diagnosketch* help patients understand their anatomy, it also gives physicians, nurses, PAs, and others the opportunity to maximize use of the very small amount of time they have with their patients. With this book at the bedside, we can be more efficient and patients leave with a better understanding of their ED visit.

—**Andrew Ulrich, MD, Professor of Emergency Medicine, Vice Chair of Operations, Yale School of Medicine**

This book is an extremely helpful tool for real-time patient education, there is really nothing available that is comparable to *Diagnosketch*. It is the best resource for concise and easy-to-understand explanations for patients of their diagnoses, while still maintaining medical accuracy and appropriate level of detail. It helps me get through to my patients and makes bedside education much smoother and more meaningful.

—**Celia Pagano, PA-C in Emergency Medicine for 6+ years**

As a nurse who spends a fair amount of time educating patients and their families, this book is a brilliant idea! It allows me the opportunity to impact patients' understanding of their disease, and is an excellent resource in triage.

—**Elizabeth Gibb, BSN, RN, Emergency Department Nurse for 41 years at the busiest EDs in New England**

I could really have used these illustrations to explain to my patient with an ovarian cyst what was going on! She was in the hospital with her dad and the doctor here was a man. I had to give the poor girl a crash course in A&P, menstruation, and explain what was going on without scaring her to death. My artwork is subpar at best, I really wish I had this book!

—**Kim Belton, RN, ER Nurse at Atrium Health with 11+ years' experience**

I use *Diagnosketch* not only with my patients at work, but also to explain my job to my children at home. It's a fantastic teaching tool!

—**Jaclyn Davis, MD, EM Physician with 10+ years' experience and Medical Staff President, Atrium Health Pineville**

I work in a rural outpatient clinic setting and make rough drawings on my own all day for patients on the paper covering the tables or the back of glove boxes. I really enjoy this book; patients find the pictures easy-to-understand and I like how clear they are.

—**Carol Venable, MD of 20+ years, EM/IM Physician, Port Townsend, WA**

This book replaces the need to pull up Google at the bedside to search for images. All common diagnoses are compiled and easy-to-understand!

—**John Burger, MD, EM Physician with 10+ years' experience in Charlotte, NC**

This book is amazing! The simplicity of it, with the wonderful illustrations, makes this an awesome teaching tool for our patients. I can't wait to share this with my team.

—**Rachel Smitek, MD, Senior Director of Quality, US Acute Care Solutions; Board-Certified Emergency Medicine doctor with 10+ years of practice**

I love this book, there are so many great visuals for the bread and butter of what we see and explain all of the time. What a great resource!

—**Katrina Barnett, MD, On Staff, El Camino Hospital, Mountain View and Los Gatos, CA; On Staff, Palo Alto VA, CA; ER physician for 15+ years**

Physicians are expected to provide excellent medical care; but it is equally important for them to explain diagnoses and treatments in a manner that gives the non-medical both understanding and reassurance. *Diagnosketch*, by emergency physician Dr. Sapana Adhikari, uses simple illustrations and text to bridge the communication gap between physician and patient so that even complex issues can be comprehended at the bedside. This will prove to be an essential tool for every emergency department.

—**Edwin Leap, MD, Emergency Physician with 30 years' experience; Columnist**

Diagnosketch

Diagnosketch:
A Visual Guide to
Medical Diagnosis for the
Non-Medical Audience

Created and Illustrated by
Sapana P. Adhikari, MD

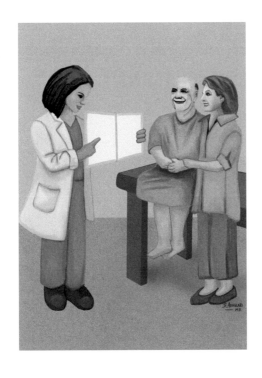

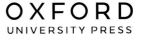

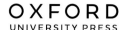

Oxford University Press is a department of the University of Oxford. It furthers the University's objective of excellence in research, scholarship, and education by publishing worldwide. Oxford is a registered trade mark of Oxford University Press in the UK and certain other countries.

Published in the United States of America by Oxford University Press
198 Madison Avenue, New York, NY 10016, United States of America.

Library of Congress Cataloging-in-Publication Data
Names: Adhikari, Sapana P., author.
Title: Diagnosketch : a visual guide to medical diagnosis for
the non-medical audience / created and illustrated by Sapana P. Adhikari.
Description: New York, NY : Oxford University Press, [2022] |
Includes bibliographical references and index. |
Identifiers: LCCN 2022012638 (print) | LCCN 2022012639 (ebook) |
ISBN 9780197636954 (paperback) | ISBN 9780197636978 (epub) |
ISBN 9780197636985 (online)
Subjects: MESH: Diagnostic Techniques and Procedures |
Medical Illustration | Health Communication—methods |
Patient Education as Topic | Critical Care | Pictorial Work
Classification: LCC RC71.3 (print) | LCC RC71.3 (ebook) | NLM WB 17 |
DDC 616.07/5—dc23/eng/20220525
LC record available at https://lccn.loc.gov/2022012638
LC ebook record available at https://lccn.loc.gov/2022012639

DOI: 10.1093/med/9780197636954.001.0001

Contents

INTRODUCTION

*D*iagnosketch is a visual aid to explain medical diagnoses to patients **at the bedside.** It uses simplified images to illustrate complicated anatomy and concepts. The title, *Diagnosketch,* combines the term "diagnosis" with the term "sketch," paralleling the way the book combines a medical diagnosis with a simplified sketch. It includes common pathologies seen in an acute care setting, especially ones that are easier to explain with pictures.

Many American patients are unfamiliar with human anatomy and common medical diagnoses. Research from the US Department of Education estimates that only 12% of English-speaking adults in the United States have proficient health literacy skills.[1] Studies indicate that almost 90% of adults have difficulty understanding health information that is currently available.[2] These patients are often unequipped to make important decisions about their own health care.

Diagnosketch improves health care literacy for the non-medical population. It simplifies human anatomy and pathophysiology into memorable, understandable images. It relies on the concept of "picture superiority effect." The picture superiority effect states that HEARING information will lead to 10% retention of the content, but HEARING and SEEING information leads to 65% retention of content. *Diagnosketch* not only explains difficult concepts to patients, but also helps patients remember them.

Diagnosketch serves as the visual guide that medical professionals use with every patient at the bedside. Excellent medical care involves diagnosing and treating disease, but just as importantly, communicating well with patients. *Diagnosketch* helps achieve this goal.

KEY COMPONENTS OF *DIAGNOSKETCH*

Simplicity

The images in the book intentionally simplify information to help educate a non-medical audience. The images leave out details that may not be clinically relevant and overemphasize those that are. Although the general anatomy is correct, certain organs are exaggerated. For example, the gallbladder is quite small in the human abdomen, yet in the images, it is depicted much larger to emphasize its clinical relevance. Also, human physiology has been simplified with colors. For example, in some images blood vessels are depicted in red whether they carry oxygenated or deoxygenated blood. In addition, the images intentionally leave out smaller anatomical structures (like nerves and smaller blood vessels) for simplicity's sake.

Practicality

The images in the book depict only the most common diagnoses seen in an acute care setting and only those that would benefit from an image. In busy settings, sometimes the health care encounter lasts just a few minutes. *Diagnosketch* presents a simple, clear image that improves understanding as quickly and efficiently as possible. In addition, the labels are minimal and are written in colloquial, non-medical language. This encourages the patient to listen to the explanation from the medical professional, rather than read and become confused by complicated medical terminology.

---

[1] Kutner, M., Greenberg, E., Jin, Y., & Paulsen, C. (2006). *The Health Literacy of America's Adults: Results From the 2003 National Assessment of Adult Literacy* (NCES 2006-483). Washington, DC: US Department of Education, National Center for Education Statistics.
[2] US Department of Health and Human Services, Office of Disease Prevention and Health Promotion. (2010). *National Action Plan to Improve Health Literacy.* Washington, DC: Author.

Inclusivity

The images in the book intentionally use various skin tones and physical features to represent the diversity seen across patients in various medical settings. Different diagnoses can affect any ethnicity. Aside from problems that affect a particular biological sex, diagnoses are depicted in the male or the female in a non-specific way.

HOW DOES *DIAGNOSKETCH* WORK?

Diagnosketch consists of 100 images of medical illnesses commonly diagnosed in an acute care setting. It is meant to be used **at the bedside** to help communicate complicated concepts to a non-medical audience quickly. Most medical encounters between doctors and patients occur verbally. Although visual aids are sometimes used, they are not standard. This book changes this paradigm by incorporating a simplified, colorful graphic visual to assist patients to better understand their diagnoses in real time.

Imagine the following scenario:

A patient presents to the emergency room for severe abdominal pain. You run tests: blood, urine, ultrasound. You diagnose cholecystitis. You **verbally** explain to your patient that her gallbladder is infected, and that she will need emergency surgery. Your patient looks dumbfounded. She never expected this. She thought that she might have eaten something bad but is now on her way to surgery? She quietly pretends that she understands but does not really know where her gallbladder is located, let alone what it does. She does not even know what questions she should ask. You sense that she does not completely understand everything, so you quickly grab a paper towel and sketch a crude image of her anatomy. Although you'd like to stay longer, you feel the pressure of a waiting room full of patients, still waiting to be seen. You rush out, knowing that although you expertly diagnosed her condition and arranged for proper treatment, you could have communicated better.

Now imagine that same patient, but this time you use *Diagnosketch*. You return to the patient's room and explain her condition verbally **AND** visually. You show your patient where her gallbladder is in relation to her other organs. You show her a gallstone and explain how it blocked her biliary tract. You show her how this caused her pain and eventually her infection. She asks pertinent questions, and you give her immediate answers. You have a two-way dialogue. In just a few minutes, you have relieved her fears and increased her anatomical knowledge. You know that you communicated in a way that she understands. When you walk out of the room, you feel confident in your skills as both a master clinician/diagnostician and, just as importantly, a master communicator.

HOW IS *DIAGNOSKETCH* ORGANIZED?

Diagnosketch is organized into seven different categories by organ systems. The categories are: skin, EENT (eye, ear, nose, throat), cardiopulmonary, gastrointestinal, genitourinary, orthopedics, and neurology. The last section, Miscellaneous, includes images that do not fit into particular organ system. There is a section on sample scripting that corresponds to each image. This section includes sample wording that serves as a starting point for better patient communication. Finally, there is an Index that includes both the medical jargon and more colloquial language a patient may use, making it easier to quickly find a particular image. Notice that on a particular image, where possible, each title is written in a colloquial language with the medical terminology listed underneath. Notice also that the labels are written in colloquial language to simplify what is happening for the non-medical patient.

Different images are helpful at different stages of a patient encounter. There are three major categories of images: diagnosis images, procedure images, and concept images.

Diagnosis images: are used to explain basic diagnoses and basic anatomy (e.g. biliary colic, kidney stone, pulmonary embolism). Many of these simplified images have a "normal" side and an "abnormal" side so that the patient can easily compare what their body part is supposed to look like with what it looks like when affected. The images also may use the "1, 2, 3 approach" that show three common problems for a particular disease (e.g. diverticulosis, diverticulitis, diverticular abscess/perforation).

Procedure images: are used to explain a procedure to a patient before performing it (e.g. IV insertion, nasogastric tube insertion, drainage of paronychia).

Concept images: are used to explain a concept visually (e.g. how to alternate ibuprofen with acetaminophen for fever reduction; how diabetes mellitus actually causes high glucose; what "code status" means).

Obviously, the images can be used in whatever way is most helpful. Here are a few real-life examples of where *Diagnosketch* has been helpful in the acute care setting:

- A nurse showed the image of "Digestion" to explain to a reluctant 10-year-old why she had to drink a bottle of contrast for an abdominal CT scan to rule out appendicitis. After the patient learned her anatomy and understood that her appendix would "light up" when she drank the contrast, she willingly drank the entire bottle without a fuss. This saved hours of time in a busy emergency room.

- A physician showed the image of "Back pain—side view" to explain the anatomy of the back to a disgruntled patient who felt that he needed an x-ray. After he understood his anatomy and why an x-ray was not indicated, he was happy to avoid unnecessary radiation exposure. This also saved the cost of an unnecessary test.

- A physician showed the image of "Urinary retention" to explain to an uncomfortable older gentleman how his enlarged prostate blocked his bladder, making it impossible to urinate. After he learned his anatomy, he felt comfortable with the insertion of the foley catheter and experienced much relief.

- A nurse showed the image of "Intravenous insertion" to her patient in the triage bay to explain how an IV works. She hoped to dispel the common misconception that an IV is a needle that stays in the arm when it is just a flexible piece of plastic.

- A physician showed the image of a "Heart attack" to the anxious male who presented with chest pain after smoking cocaine. After he visually saw how cocaine could cause his heart muscle to die, he vowed to never use it again. This potentially deterred future drug usage.

HOW DO PATIENTS FEEL AFTER SEEING *DIAGNOSKETCH*?

Patients often ask for a copy of the *Diagnosketch* image to take home. Sometimes, they take a picture on their cell phone to explain to their family members later. Many patients have access to the internet at home and can extensively research their diagnosis. Yet, once they leave the hospital, they almost always do not. Instead, they rely on the simple, familiar images that the medical professional explained to them that they understand.

There are many beautiful anatomy books available with detailed pictures. There are hundreds of images on the internet about anatomy and diagnoses. There is helpful information on discharge paperwork from a hospital or clinic. Diagnosketch does not try to compete with these very useful resources. Instead, it serves as the first basic primer to understanding the medical diagnosis. Once the medical encounter ends, the patient is now equipped with solid knowledge of basic anatomy and physiology and encouraged to further investigate more complicated medical information.

Diagnosketch is a quick, useful tool that greatly enhances the patient's experience. All images are in one place. All images are at a simplistic level of detail. And, all images are clinically useful and relevant to the medical problem at hand.

ABOUT THE AUTHOR/ILLUSTRATOR

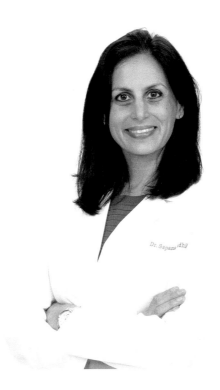

I have worked as an emergency medicine physician for 20 years and have seen poor health literacy affect my patients firsthand. For this reason, I developed *Diagnosketch*. I believe that each patient deserves customized knowledge about their anatomy and pathology relevant to their health care encounter.

Early in my career, I drew stick figures and anatomy on paper towels or on whiteboards in my patients' rooms. I saw the utility of visual aids to explain medical concepts. Over the years, I created better images that incorporated real-time patient feedback. I tried many different iterations: everything from more realistic, traditional images to super "cartoony" images. I found that the perfect style of illustration lies between the two. The style in *Diagnosketch* works best because it relays accurate information in a simple, colorful, and non-threatening way. It gets the point across without being too cartoony or "dumbed down." I now use these images with the majority of my patients. It is satisfying to know

that I have not only treated diseases but also helped my patients understand their diagnoses.

I realized that we, as medical professionals, do a great job diagnosing disease. We run blood tests, urine tests, x-rays, and CT scans. We come up with an accurate diagnosis and start proper treatments. Yet, sometimes, when we try to explain everything to our patients, we may not communicate the information as clearly as possible. I hope that *Diagnosketch* will be used to fill this gap.

Diagnosketch is a multiyear project with multiple revisions and rounds of feedback. I welcome your suggestions, comments, and feedback to make it a useful tool for all patient education needs. Thank you.

Sapana Adhikari, MD
https://www.diagnosketch.com
diagnosketch@gmail.com

SKIN

BLOOD DRAW

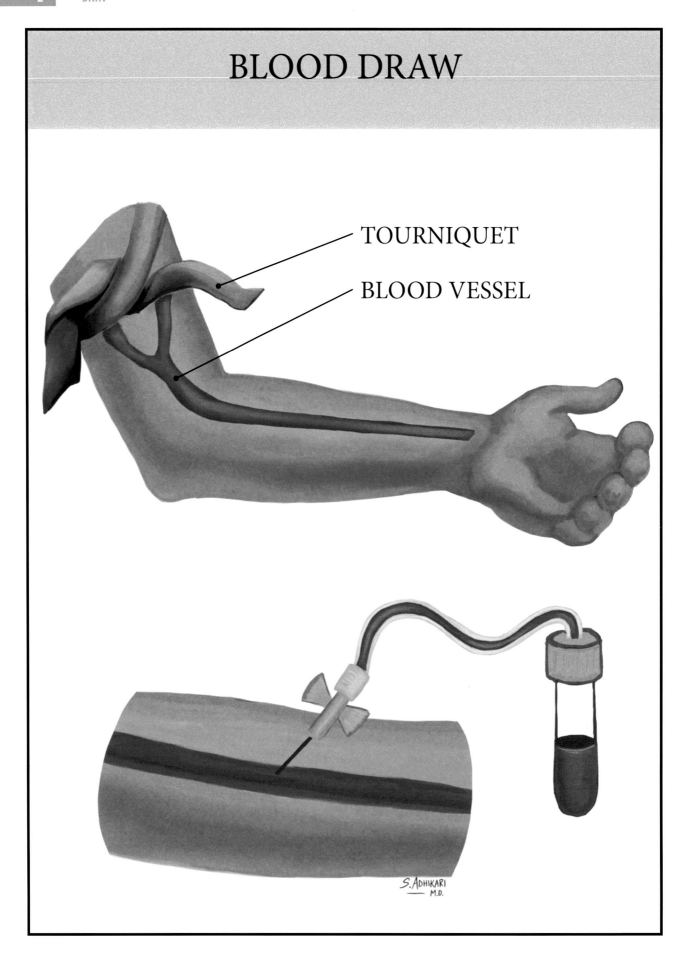

TOURNIQUET

BLOOD VESSEL

S. ADHIKARI
M.D.

IV
INTRAVENOUS INSERTION

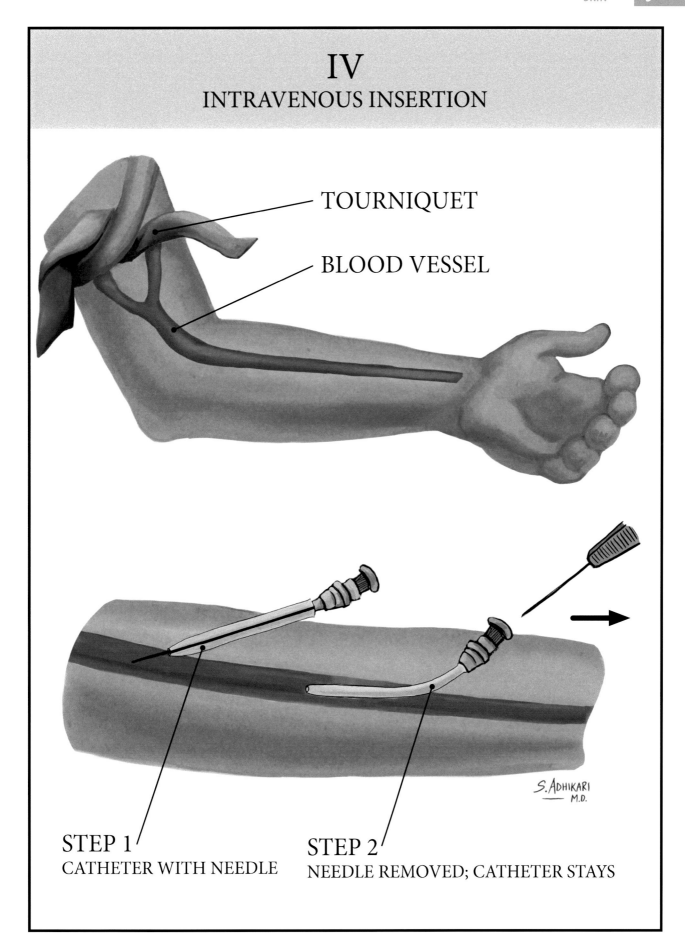

TOURNIQUET

BLOOD VESSEL

S. ADHIKARI
M.D.

STEP 1
CATHETER WITH NEEDLE

STEP 2
NEEDLE REMOVED; CATHETER STAYS

CUT
LACERATION

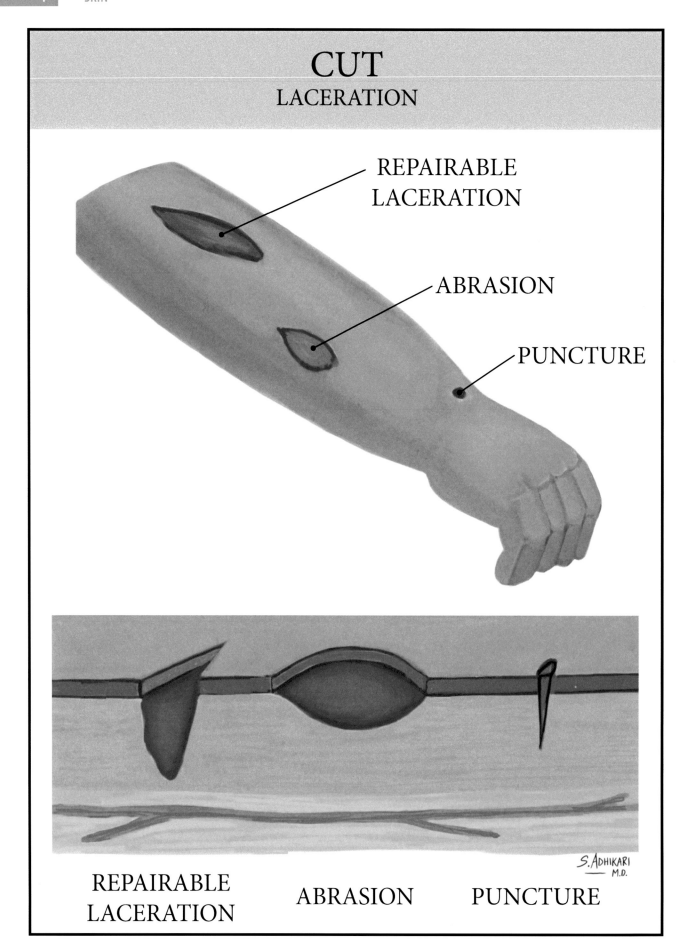

REPAIRABLE
LACERATION

ABRASION

PUNCTURE

S. ADHIKARI
M.D.

REPAIRABLE
LACERATION

ABRASION

PUNCTURE

OPTIONS FOR REPAIR

LACERATION

ABRASION

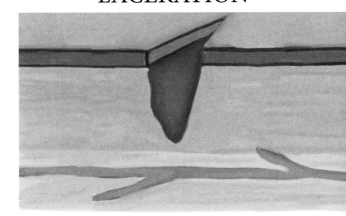

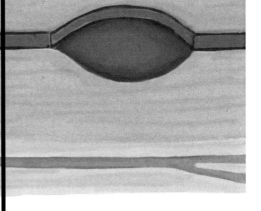

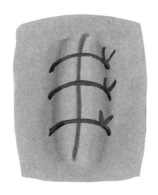

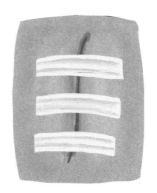

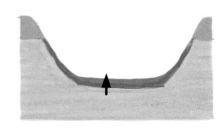

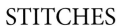 STITCHES

STERI-STRIPS

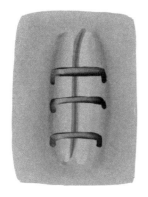

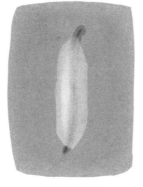

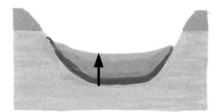

STAPLES

GLUE

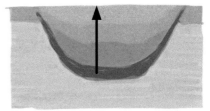

FILLS IN

S. Adhikari M.D.

BOIL
ABSCESS

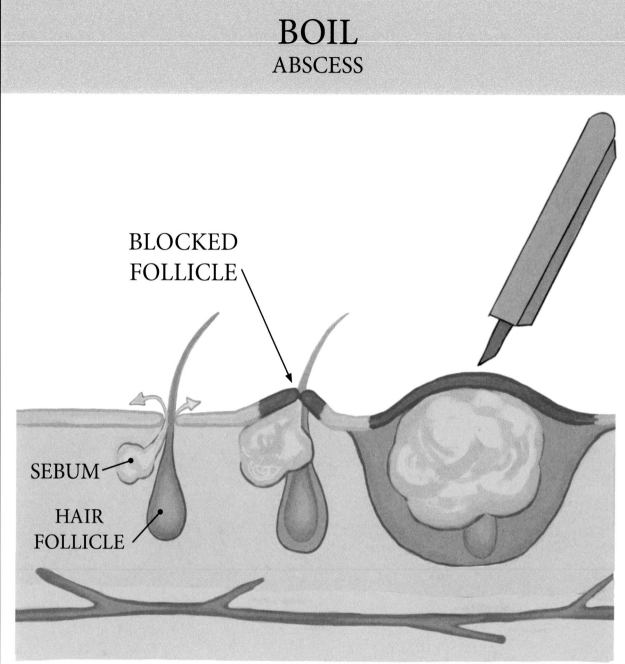

BLOCKED
FOLLICLE

SEBUM

HAIR
FOLLICLE

S. ADHIKARI
M.D.

NORMAL

EARLY
ABSCESS

LATE
ABSCESS

MRSA
METHICILLIN-RESISTANT *STAPHYLOCOCCUS AUREUS*

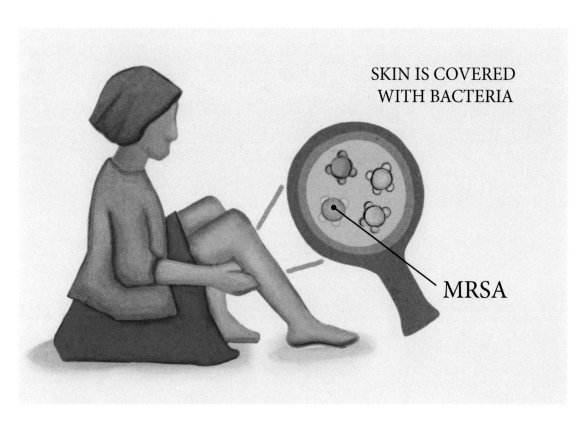

SKIN IS COVERED
WITH BACTERIA

MRSA

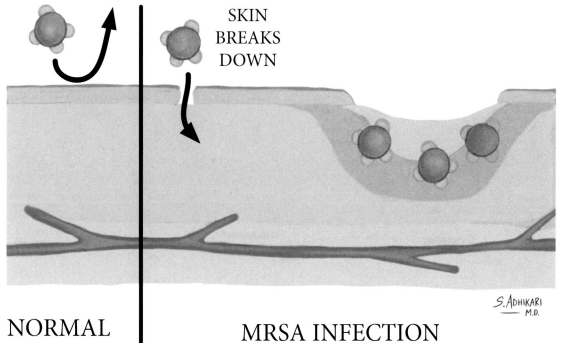

SKIN
BREAKS
DOWN

S. ADHIKARI
M.D.

NORMAL

MRSA INFECTION

PARONYCHIA

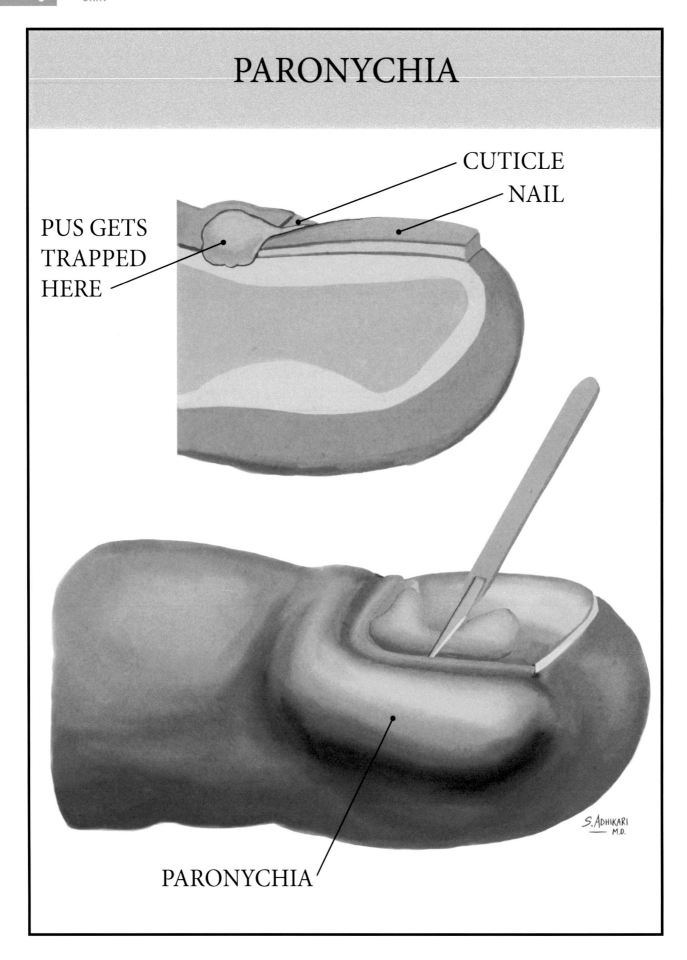

CUTICLE

NAIL

PUS GETS
TRAPPED
HERE

PARONYCHIA

CRUSHED FINGER
SUBUNGUAL HEMATOMA

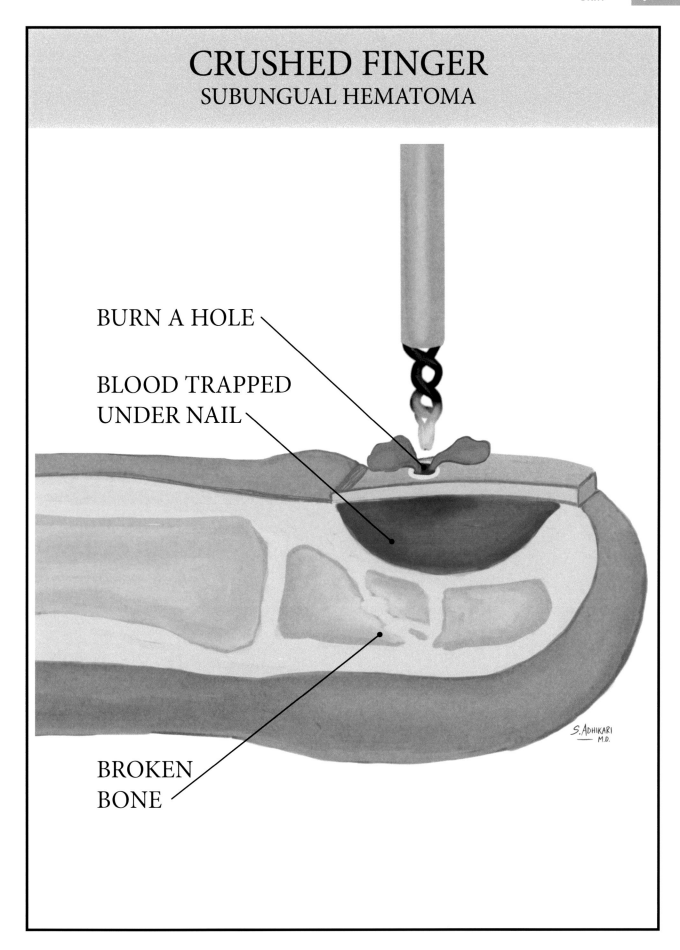

BURN A HOLE

BLOOD TRAPPED
UNDER NAIL

BROKEN
BONE

S. ADHIKARI
M.D.

SUPERFICIAL CLOT
SUPERFICIAL THROMBOPHLEBITIS

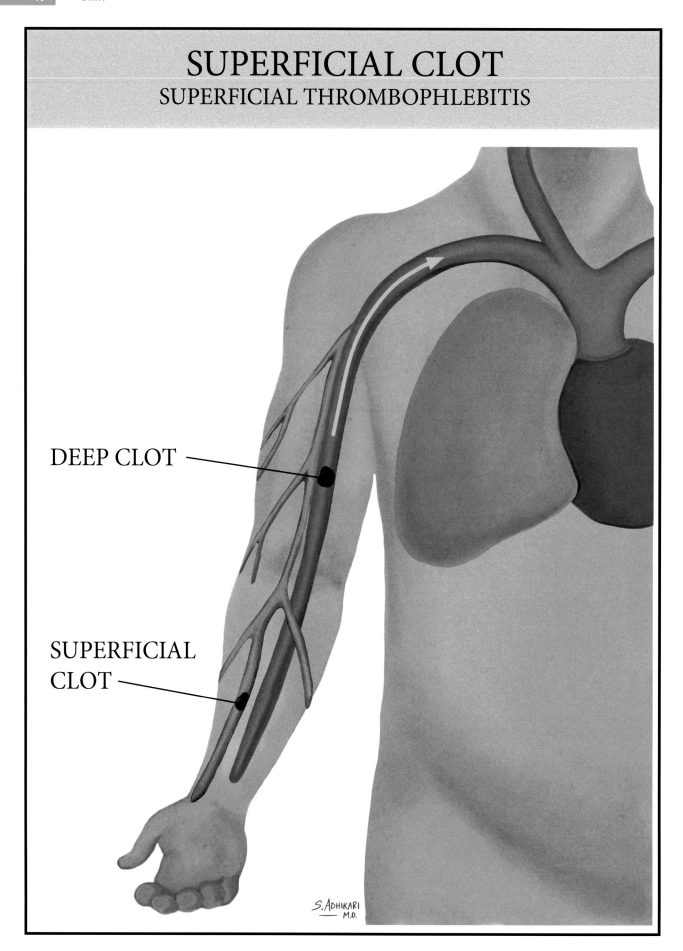

DEEP CLOT

SUPERFICIAL
CLOT

S. ADHIKARI
M.D.

AIRWAY ANATOMY

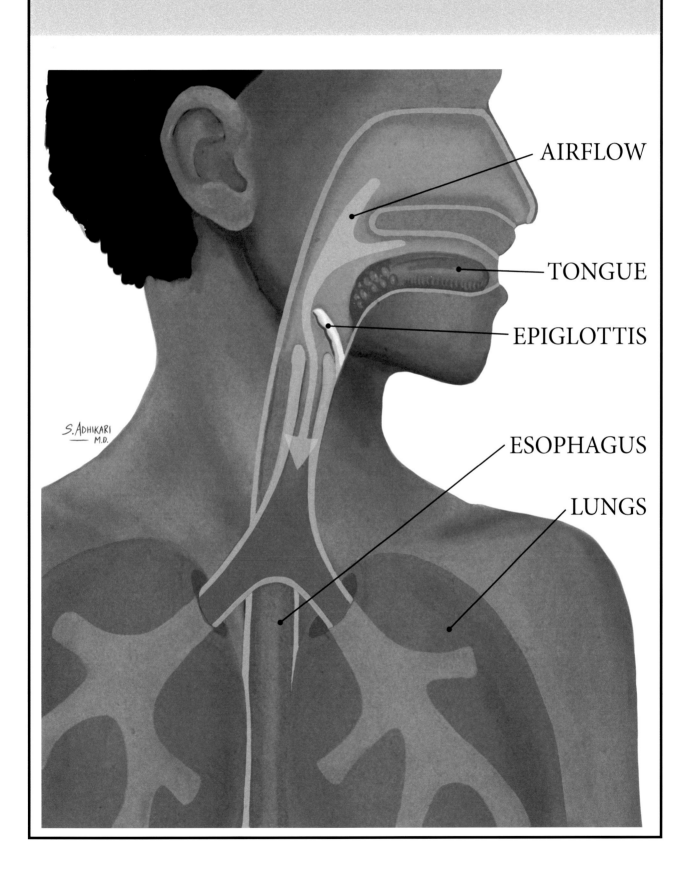

AIRFLOW

TONGUE

EPIGLOTTIS

ESOPHAGUS

LUNGS

EENT (EYE, EAR, NOSE, THROAT)

EYE PAIN
CORNEAL ABRASION & CONJUNCTIVITIS

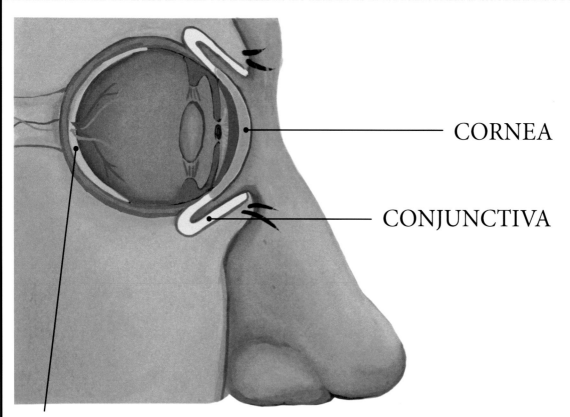

CORNEA

CONJUNCTIVA

RETINA

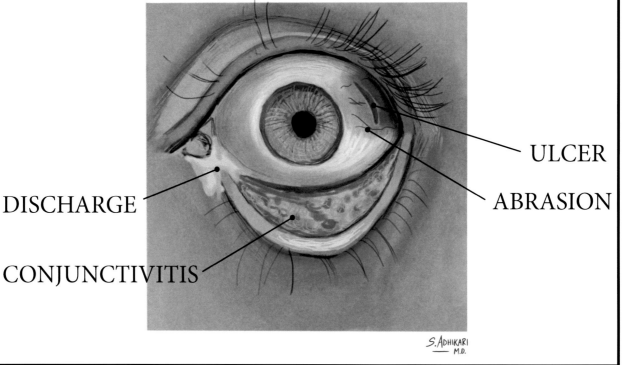

ULCER

DISCHARGE

ABRASION

CONJUNCTIVITIS

S. ADHIKARI
M.D.

TOOTHACHE
DENTAL CARIES vs DENTAL ABSCESS

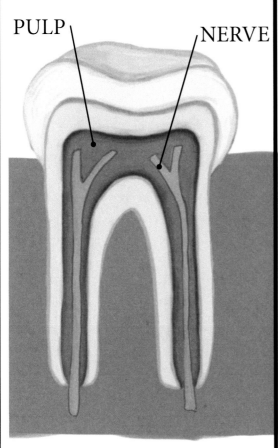

PULP   NERVE

NORMAL

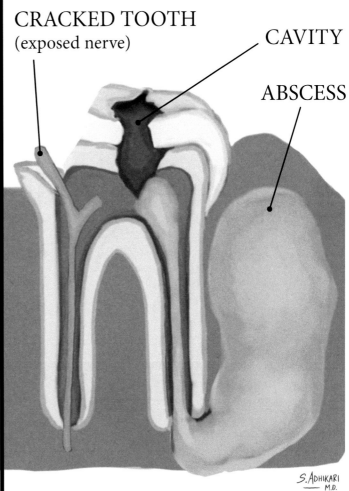

CRACKED TOOTH
(exposed nerve)

CAVITY

ABSCESS

S. ADHIKARI
M.D.

TOOTHACHE

NOSEBLEED
EPISTAXIS

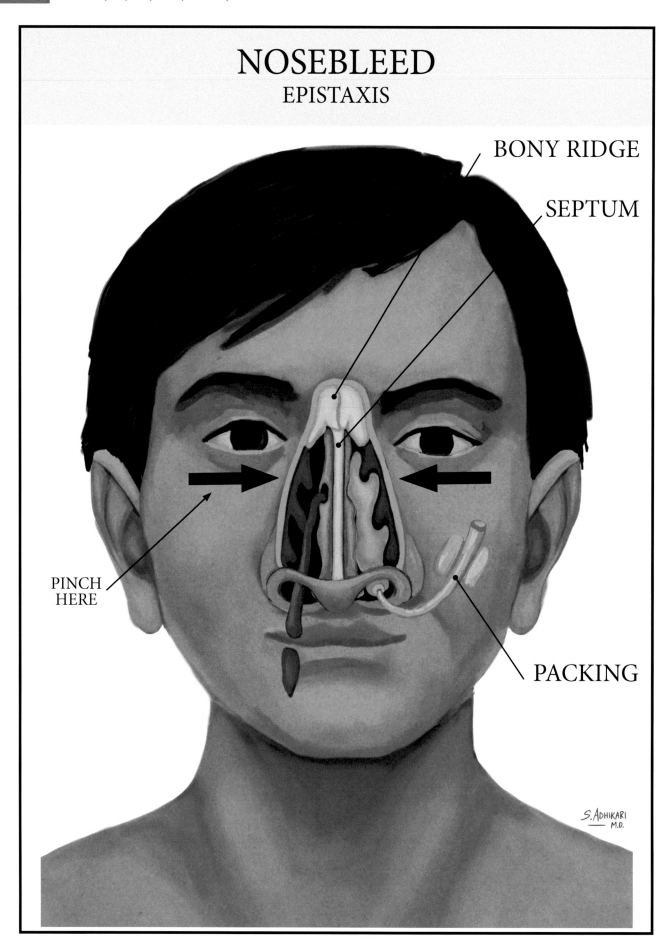

BONY RIDGE

SEPTUM

PINCH
HERE

PACKING

S. ADHIKARI
M.D.

SINUS INFECTION
SINUSITIS

NORMAL   SINUSITIS

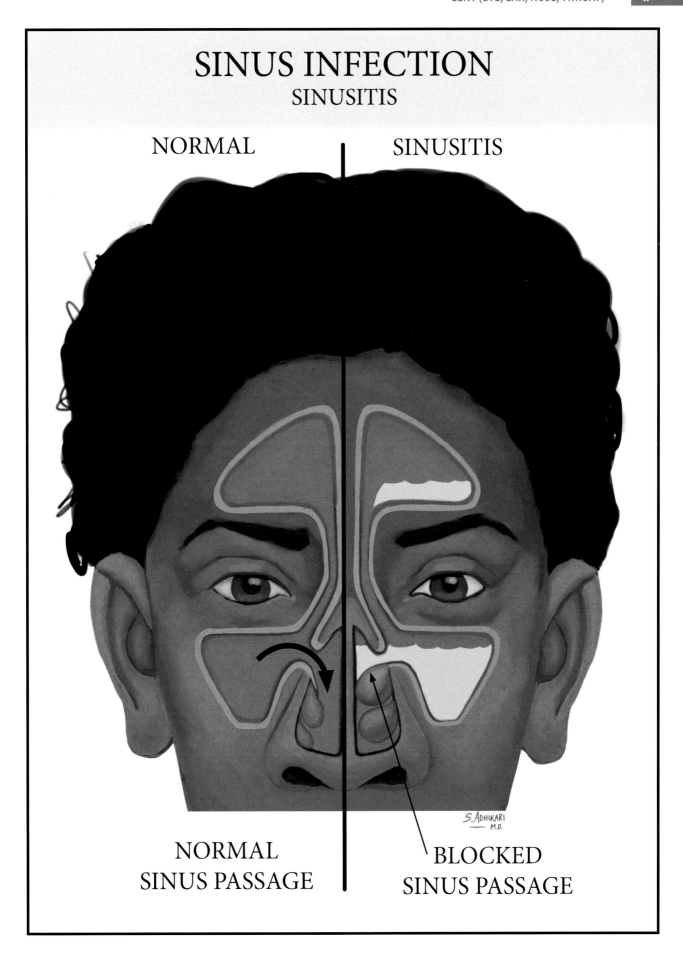

NORMAL
SINUS PASSAGE

BLOCKED
SINUS PASSAGE

S. ADHIKARI
M.D.

INNER EAR INFECTION
OTITIS MEDIA

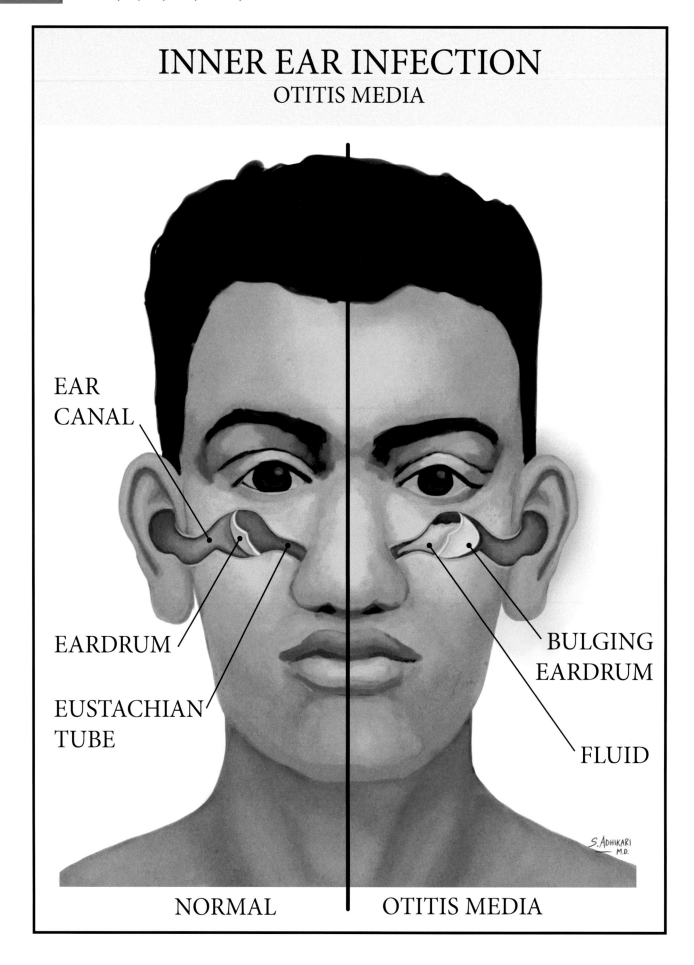

EAR
CANAL

EARDRUM

EUSTACHIAN
TUBE

BULGING
EARDRUM

FLUID

NORMAL   OTITIS MEDIA

SWIMMER'S EAR
OTITIS EXTERNA

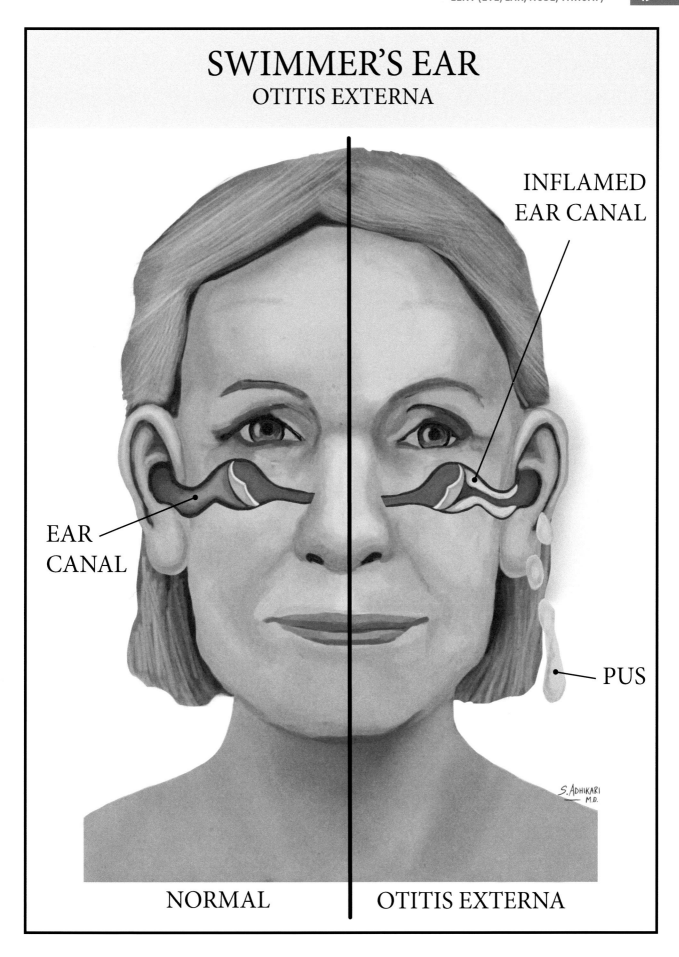

INFLAMED
EAR CANAL

EAR
CANAL

PUS

NORMAL | OTITIS EXTERNA

SORE THROAT
STREP PHARYNGITIS & PERITONSILLAR ABSCESS (PTA)

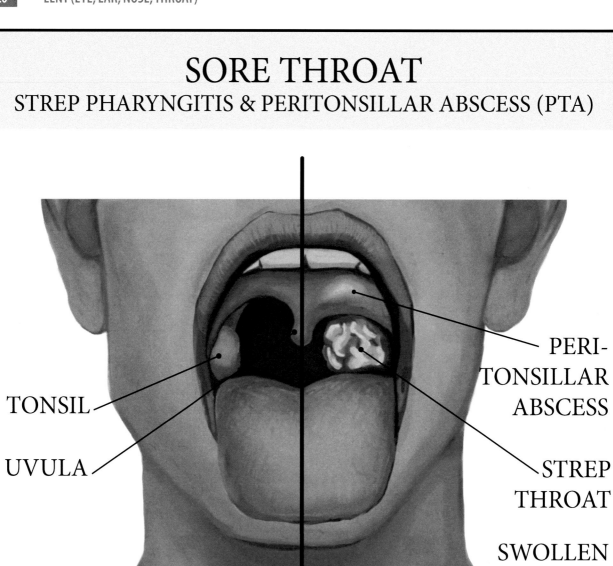

TONSIL

UVULA

PERI-
TONSILLAR
ABSCESS

STREP
THROAT

SWOLLEN
LYMPH NODE

S. ADHIKARI
M.D.

NORMAL   SORE THROAT

CARDIOPULMONARY

BRONCHITIS vs PNEUMONIA

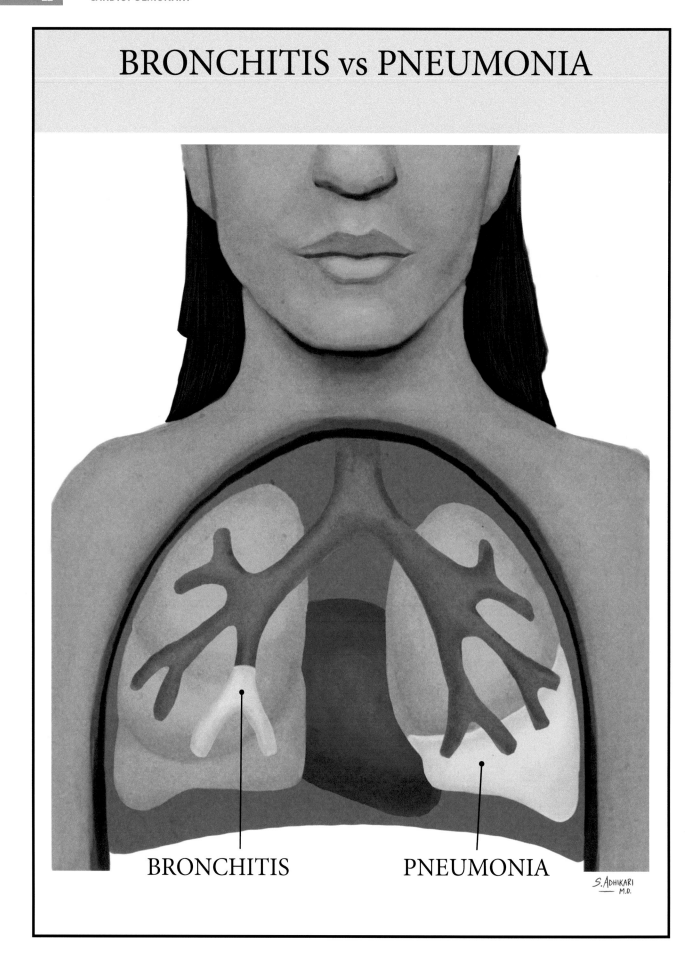

BRONCHITIS   PNEUMONIA

S. ADHIKARI
M.D.

EMPHYSEMA
CHRONIC OBSTRUCTIVE PULMONARY DISEASE (COPD)

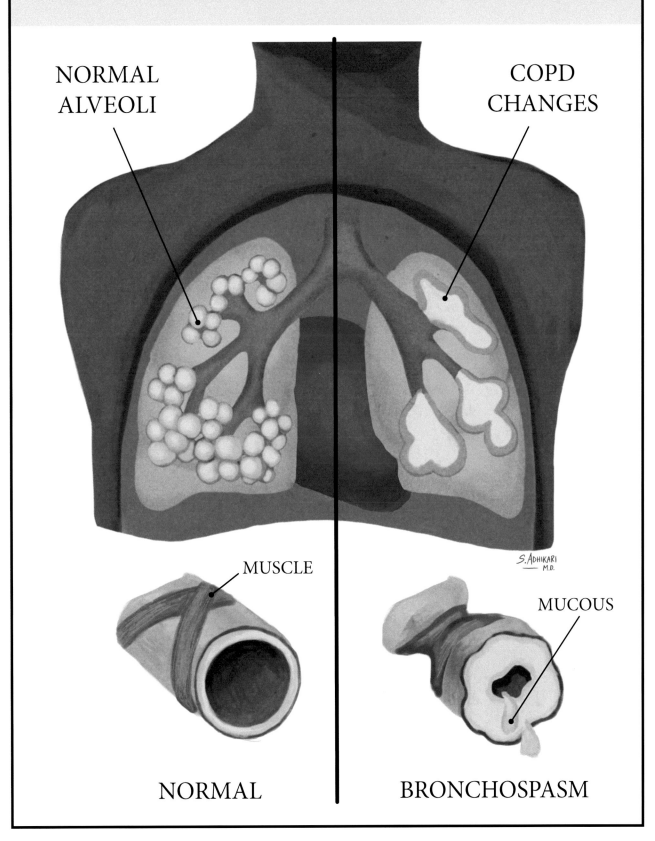

NORMAL
ALVEOLI

COPD
CHANGES

MUSCLE

MUCOUS

S. ADHIKARI
M.D.

NORMAL

BRONCHOSPASM

BLOOD CLOT
DEEP VEIN THROMBOSIS (DVT) & PULMONARY EMBOLISM (PE)

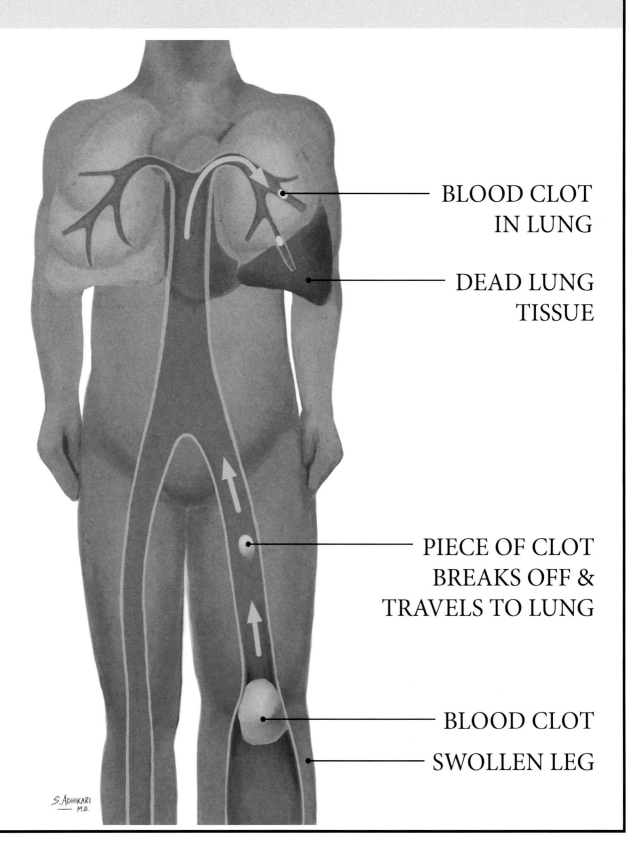

BLOOD CLOT
IN LUNG

DEAD LUNG
TISSUE

PIECE OF CLOT
BREAKS OFF &
TRAVELS TO LUNG

BLOOD CLOT

SWOLLEN LEG

S. ADHIKARI
M.D.

SWOLLEN LEGS
PEDAL EDEMA

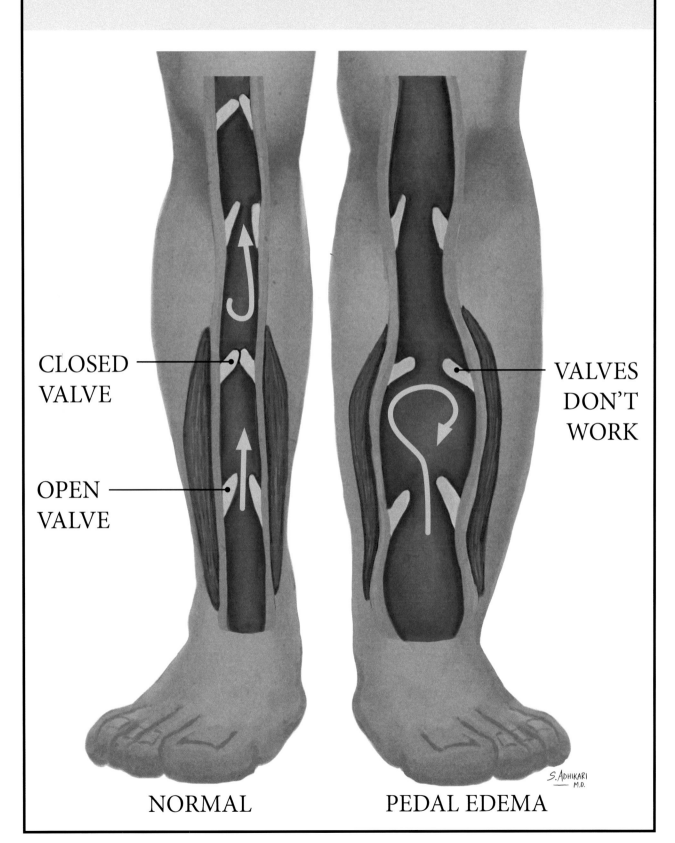

CLOSED
VALVE

OPEN
VALVE

VALVES
DON'T
WORK

S. ADHIKARI
M.D.

NORMAL   PEDAL EDEMA

HEART ATTACK
MYOCARDIAL INFARCTION (MI)

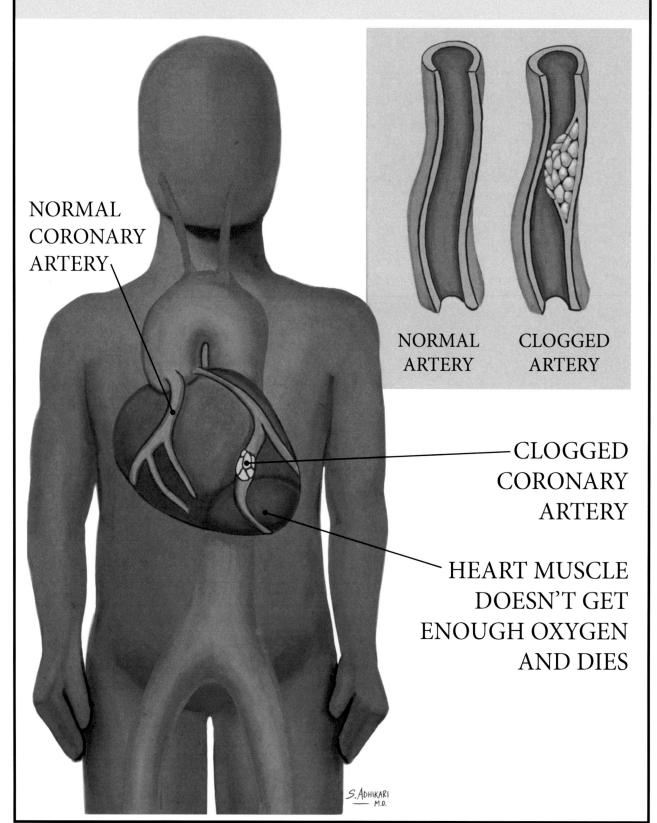

NORMAL
CORONARY
ARTERY

NORMAL
ARTERY

CLOGGED
ARTERY

CLOGGED
CORONARY
ARTERY

HEART MUSCLE
DOESN'T GET
ENOUGH OXYGEN
AND DIES

S. ADHIKARI
M.D.

CHEST PAIN EVALUATION

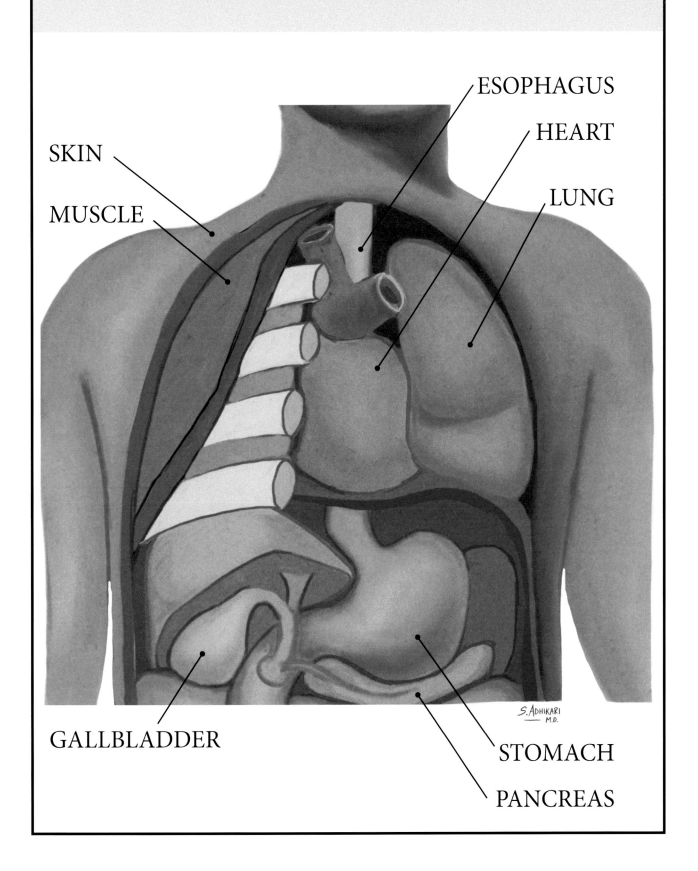

ESOPHAGUS

HEART

LUNG

SKIN

MUSCLE

GALLBLADDER

STOMACH

PANCREAS

S. ADHIKARI
M.D.

HEART FAILURE
CONGESTIVE HEART FAILURE (CHF)

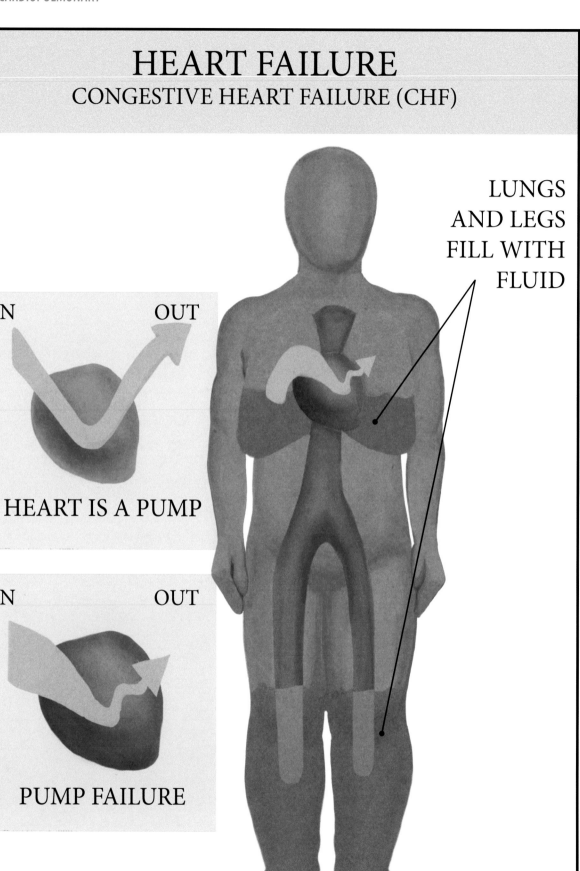

IN   OUT

HEART IS A PUMP

IN   OUT

PUMP FAILURE

LUNGS
AND LEGS
FILL WITH
FLUID

S. ADHIKARI
M.D.

HEART FAILURE CAUSES
DIASTOLIC vs SYSTOLIC DISEASE

DIASTOLIC
DISEASE

SYSTOLIC
DISEASE

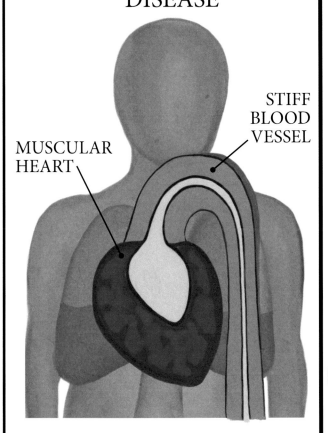

MUSCULAR
HEART

STIFF
BLOOD
VESSEL

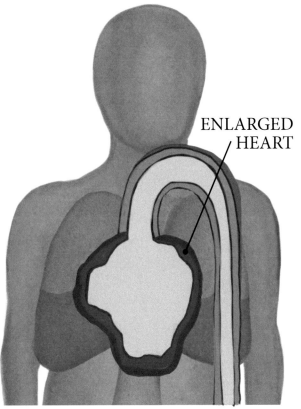

ENLARGED
HEART

S. ADHIKARI
M.D.

HEART CANNOT
PUMP AGAINST STIFF
BLOOD VESSELS

ENLARGED HEART IS
TOO WEAK TO PUMP

HIGH BLOOD PRESSURE
HYPERTENSION (HTN)

NORMAL

HTN

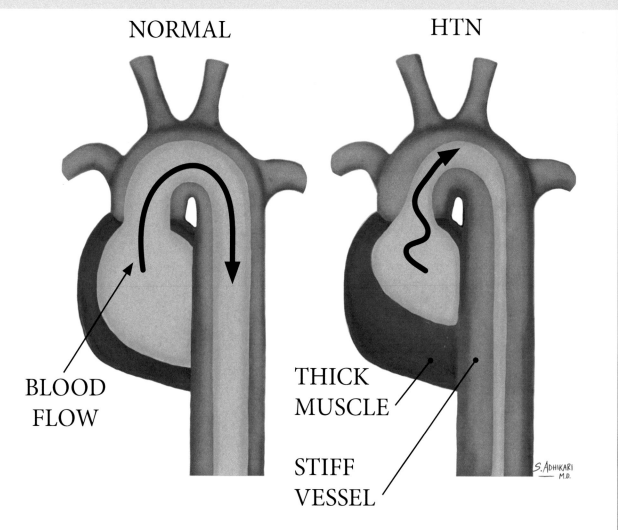

BLOOD
FLOW

THICK
MUSCLE

STIFF
VESSEL

S. ADHIKARI
M.D.

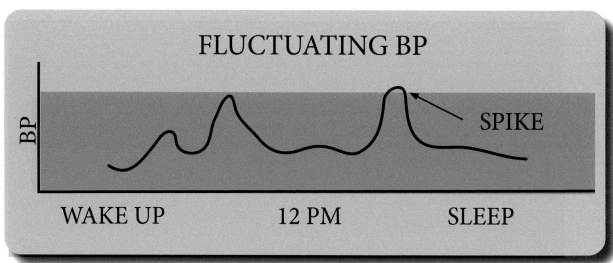

FLUCTUATING BP

BP

SPIKE

WAKE UP   12 PM   SLEEP

HTN + SYMPTOMS
HYPERTENSIVE URGENCY

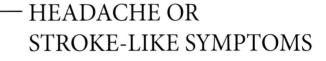

HEADACHE OR
STROKE-LIKE SYMPTOMS

CHEST PAIN

SHORTNESS OF BREATH

ABDOMINAL PAIN

BACK PAIN

POOR CIRCULATION

S. ADHIKARI
M.D.

IRREGULAR HEART BEAT
ATRIAL FIBRILLATION

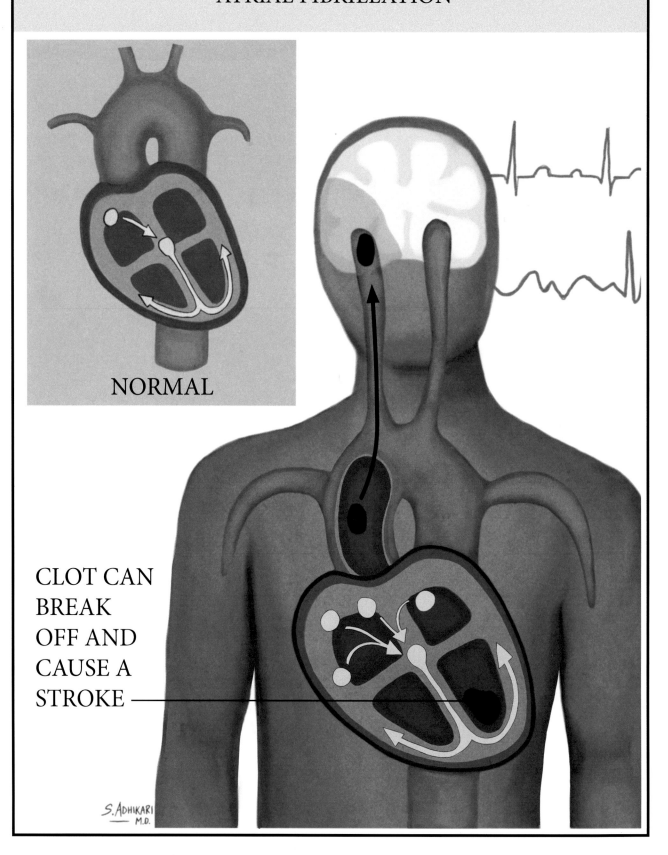

NORMAL

CLOT CAN
BREAK
OFF AND
CAUSE A
STROKE —

S. ADHIKARI
M.D.

FLUID AROUND HEART
PERICARDITIS vs PERICARDIAL EFFUSION

NORMAL

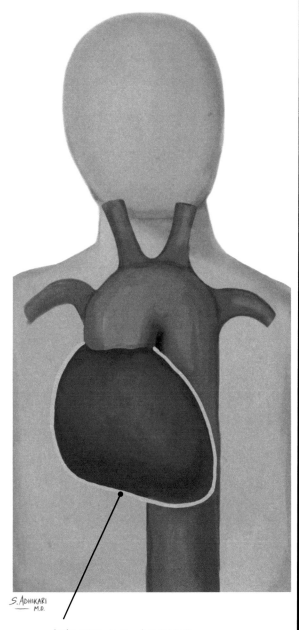

THIN LAYER
AROUND HEART

FLUID AROUND HEART

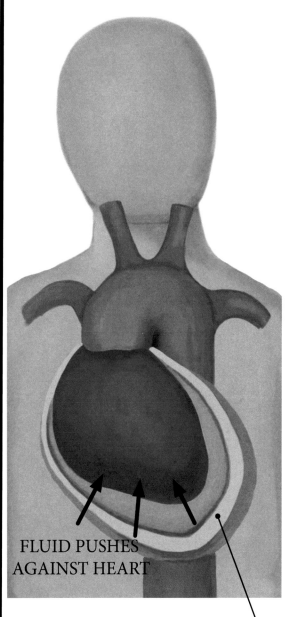

FLUID PUSHES
AGAINST HEART

INFLAMED LAYER
AROUND HEART

AORTIC DISSECTION

AORTA

HEART

TEAR IN
THE WALL
OF THE
AORTA

S. ADHIKARI
M.D.

AORTIC ANEURYSM

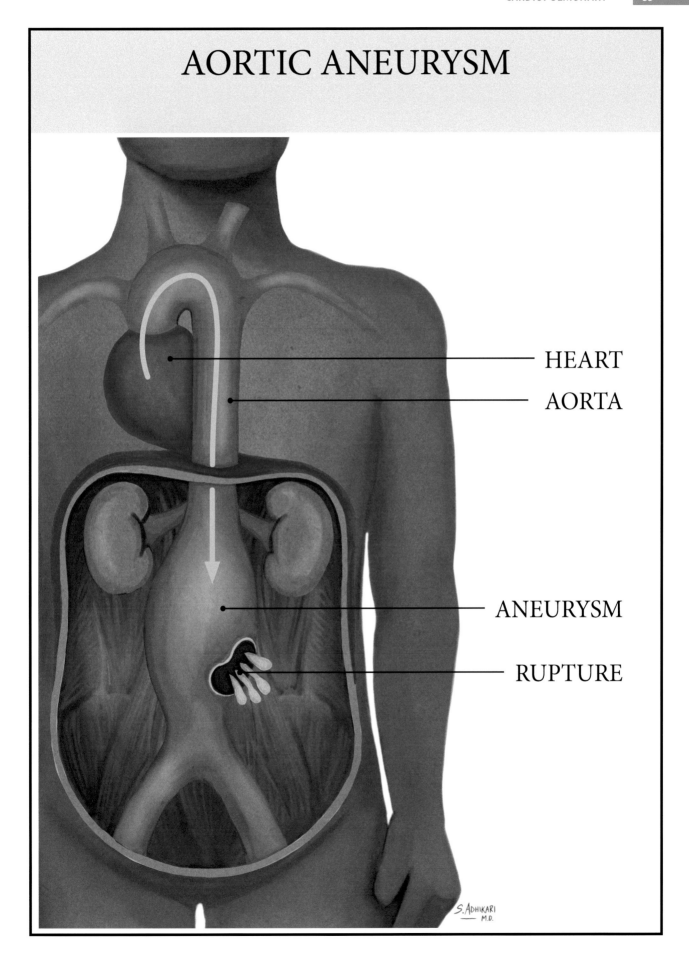

HEART

AORTA

ANEURYSM

RUPTURE

S. ADHIKARI
M.D.

POOR CIRCULATION
PERIPHERAL ARTERY DISEASE & VENOUS INSUFFICIENCY

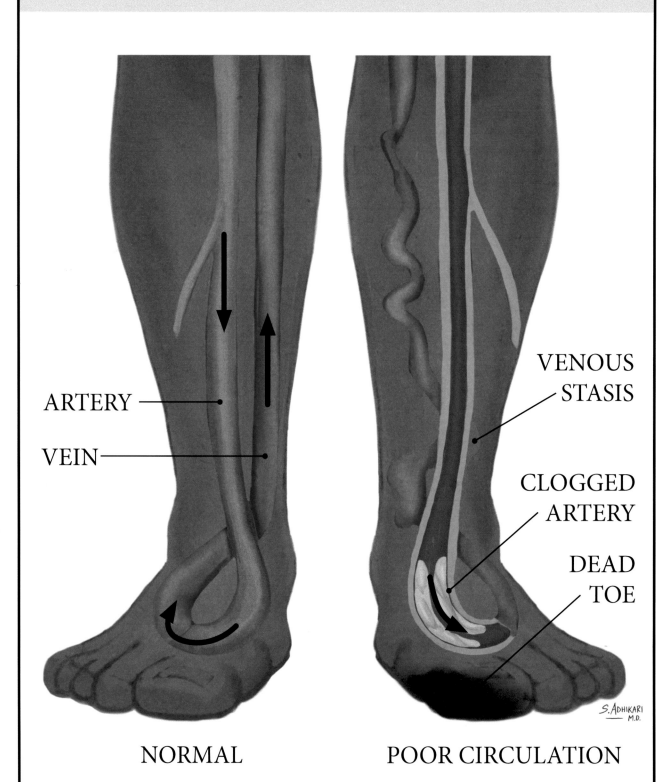

ARTERY

VEIN

VENOUS STASIS

CLOGGED ARTERY

DEAD TOE

S. ADHIKARI M.D.

NORMAL

POOR CIRCULATION

GASTROINTESTINAL

DIGESTION

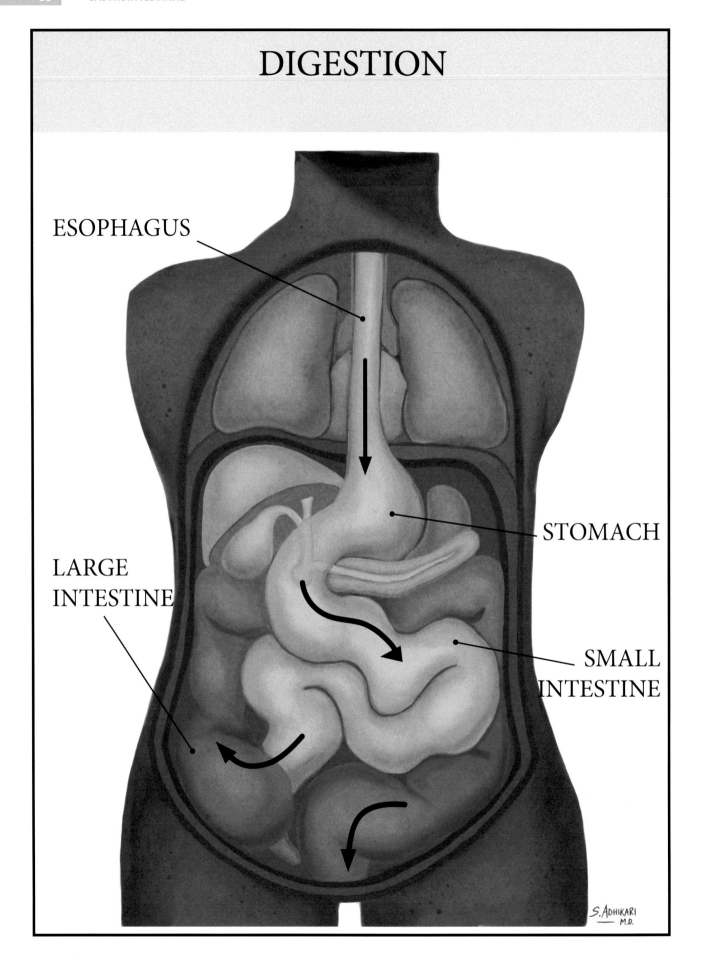

ESOPHAGUS

STOMACH

LARGE
INTESTINE

SMALL
INTESTINE

S. ADHIKARI
M.D.

ABDOMINAL PAIN

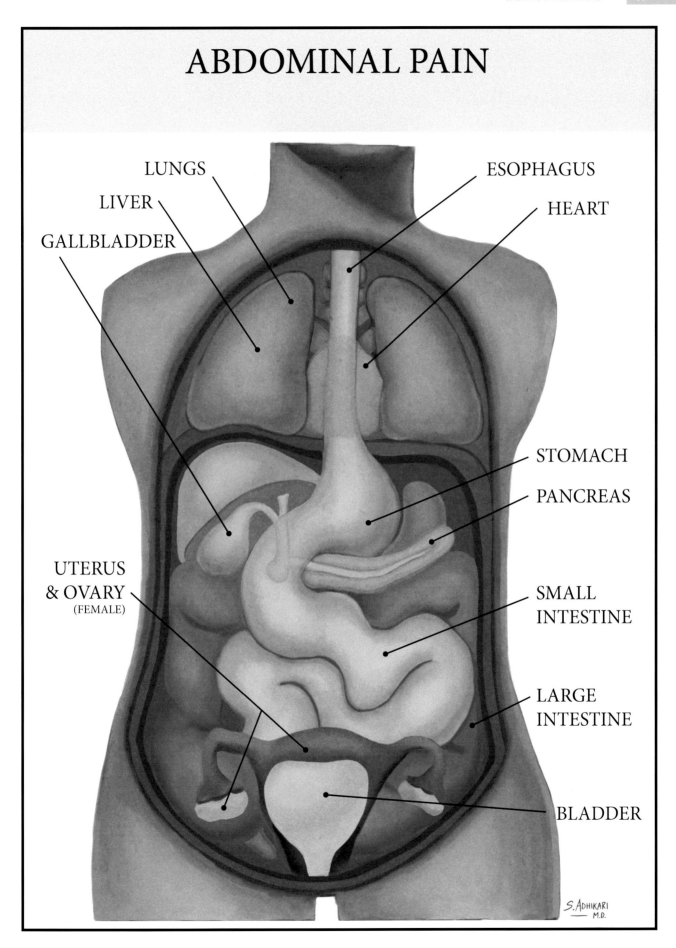

LUNGS

LIVER

GALLBLADDER

ESOPHAGUS

HEART

STOMACH

PANCREAS

UTERUS
& OVARY
(FEMALE)

SMALL
INTESTINE

LARGE
INTESTINE

BLADDER

S. Adhikari
M.D.

HEARTBURN
GASTROESOPHAGEAL REFLUX DISEASE (GERD)

SPHINCTER
CLOSED

SPHINCTER
OPEN

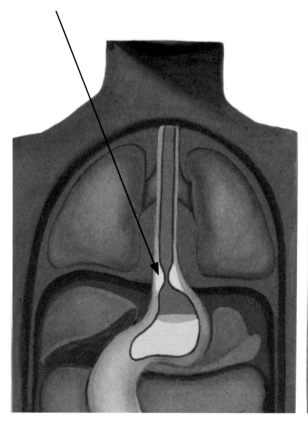

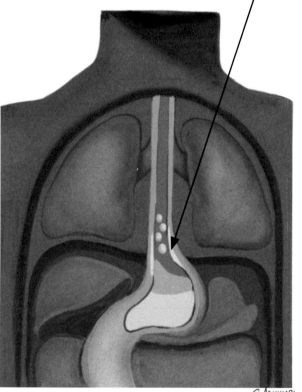

NORMAL
ACID STAYS IN
THE STOMACH

HEARTBURN
ACID BURNS
ESOPHAGUS

GASTRITIS & ULCER

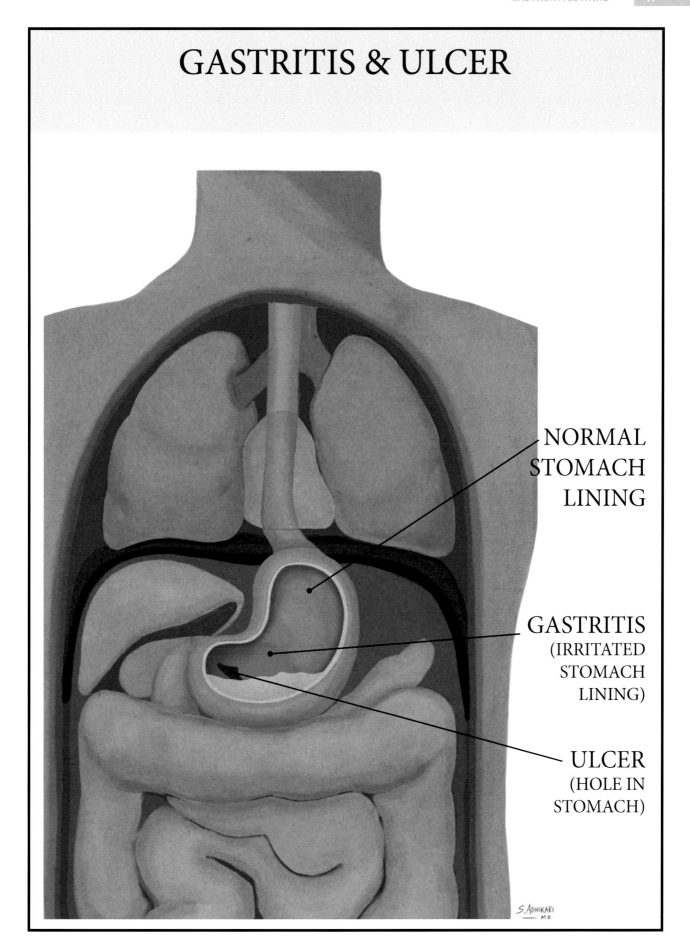

NORMAL
STOMACH
LINING

GASTRITIS
(IRRITATED
STOMACH
LINING)

ULCER
(HOLE IN
STOMACH)

S. ADHIKARI
M D

VOMITING BLOOD
UPPER GASTROINTESTINAL BLEED (UGIB)

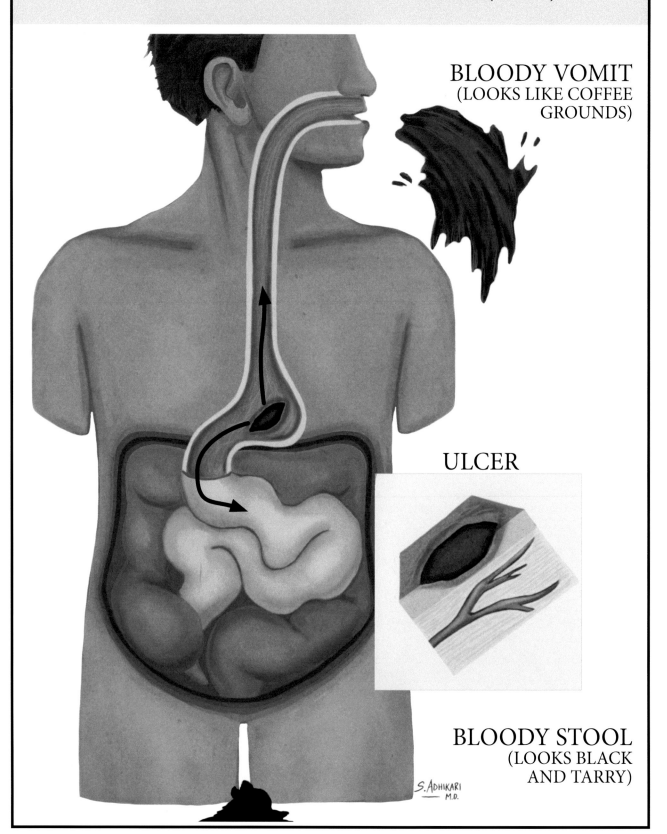

BLOODY VOMIT
(LOOKS LIKE COFFEE
GROUNDS)

ULCER

BLOODY STOOL
(LOOKS BLACK
AND TARRY)

S. ADHIKARI
M.D.

RECTAL BLEED
LOWER GASTROINTESTINAL BLEED (LGIB)

AVM
(ARTERIO-VENOUS MALFORMATION)

DIVERTICULAR
BLEED

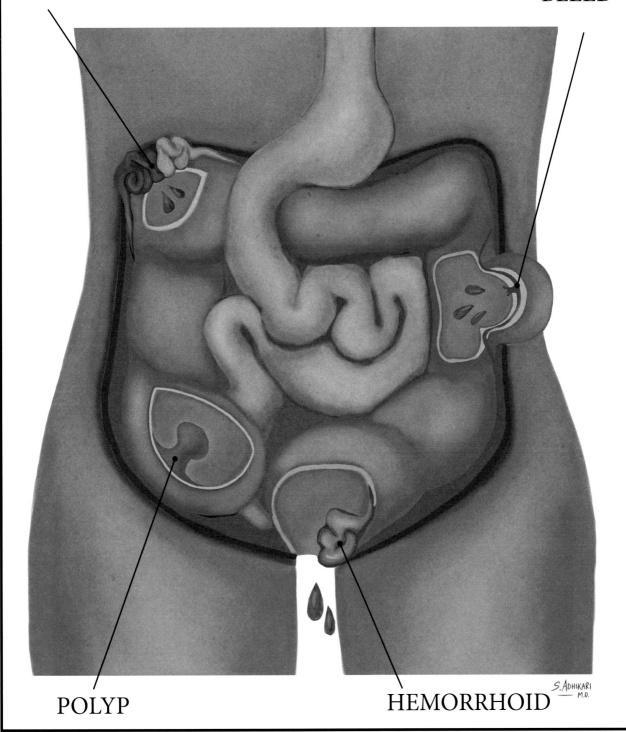

POLYP

HEMORRHOID

S.ADHIKARI
M.D.

HIATAL HERNIA

NORMAL

HIATAL HERNIA

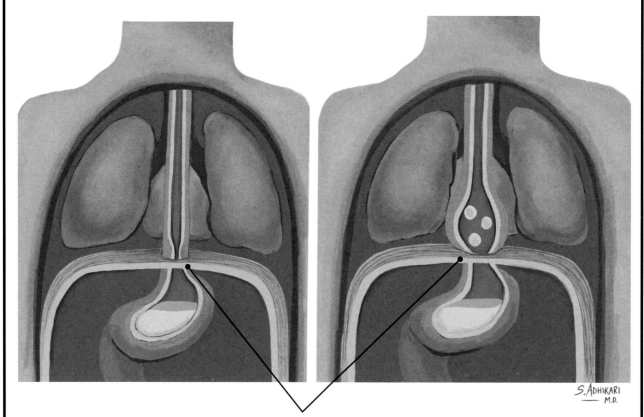

DIAPHRAGM

HERNIA
NORMAL vs INCARCERATED

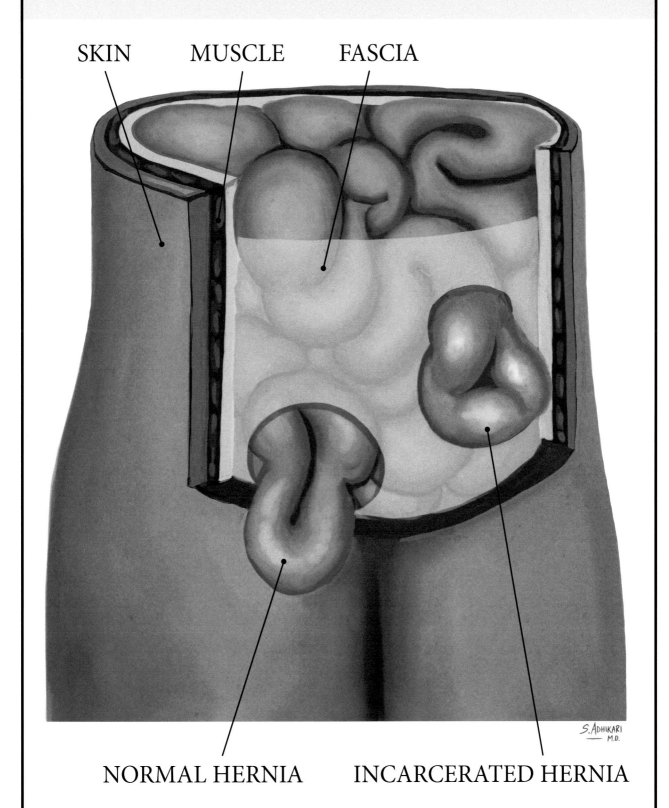

SKIN MUSCLE FASCIA

NORMAL HERNIA INCARCERATED HERNIA

FOREIGN BODY IN ESOPHAGUS
ESOPHAGEAL STRICTURE

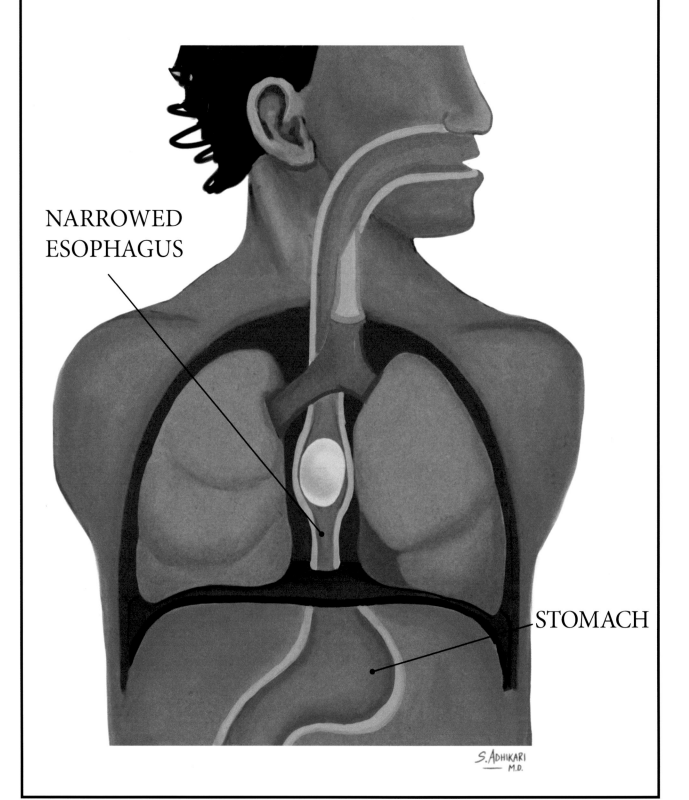

NARROWED
ESOPHAGUS

STOMACH

S. ADHIKARI
M.D.

BOWEL BLOCKAGE
SMALL BOWEL OBSTRUCTION (SBO)

NASO-GASTRIC TUBE

OBSTRUCTION

S. ADHIKARI
M.D.

GALLBLADDER DISEASE
BILIARY COLIC

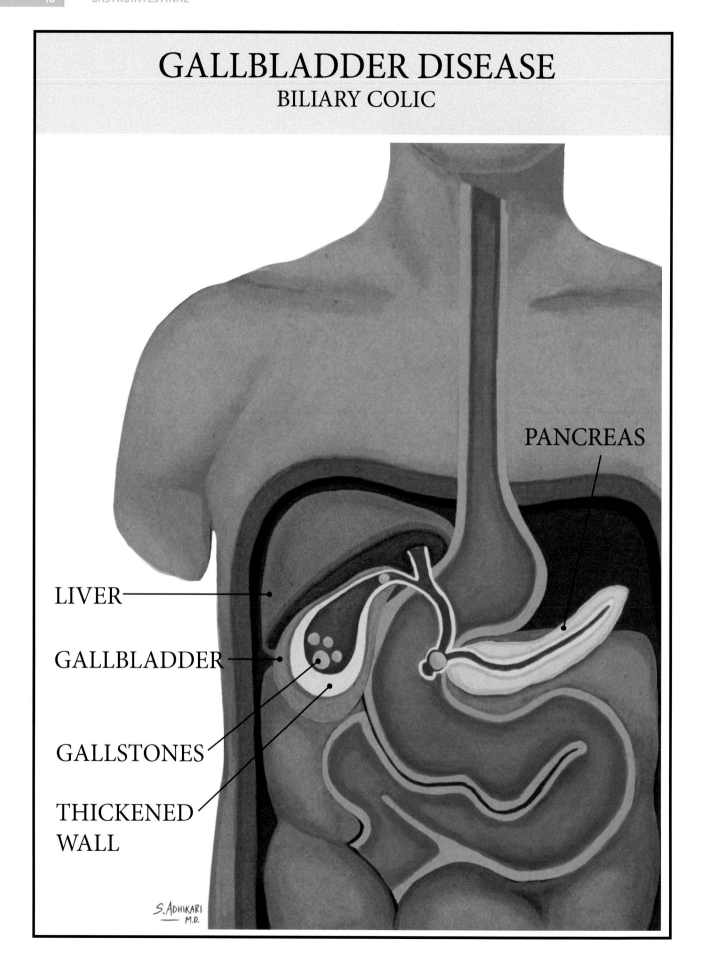

PANCREAS

LIVER

GALLBLADDER

GALLSTONES

THICKENED
WALL

S. ADHIKARI
M.D.

PANCREATITIS

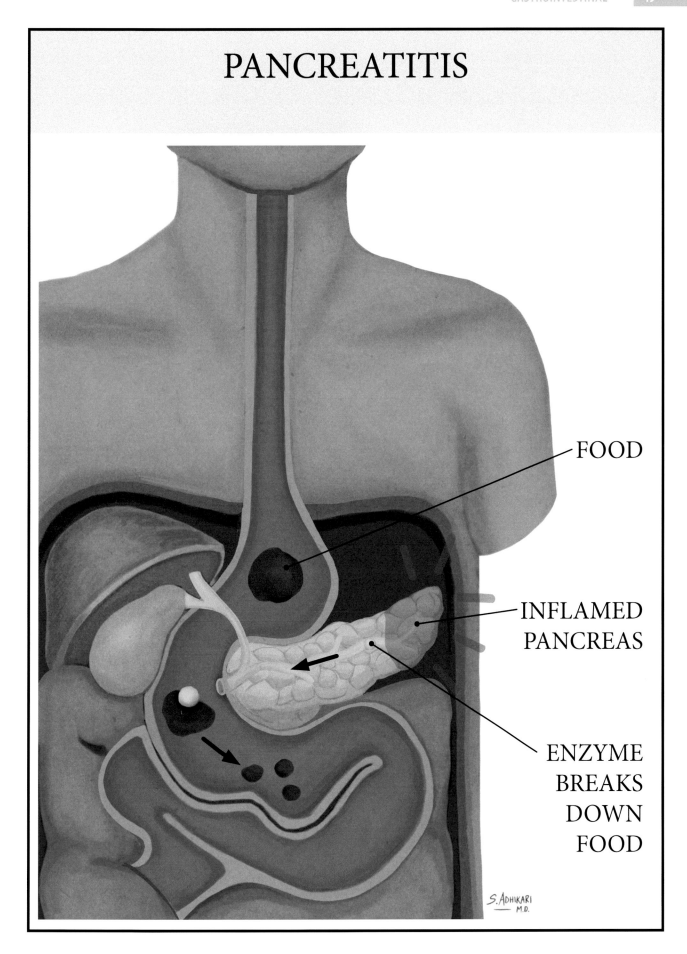

FOOD

INFLAMED PANCREAS

ENZYME BREAKS DOWN FOOD

S. ADHIKARI M.D.

DIVERTICULAR DISEASE
DIVERTICULOSIS, DIVERTICULITIS & PERFORATION

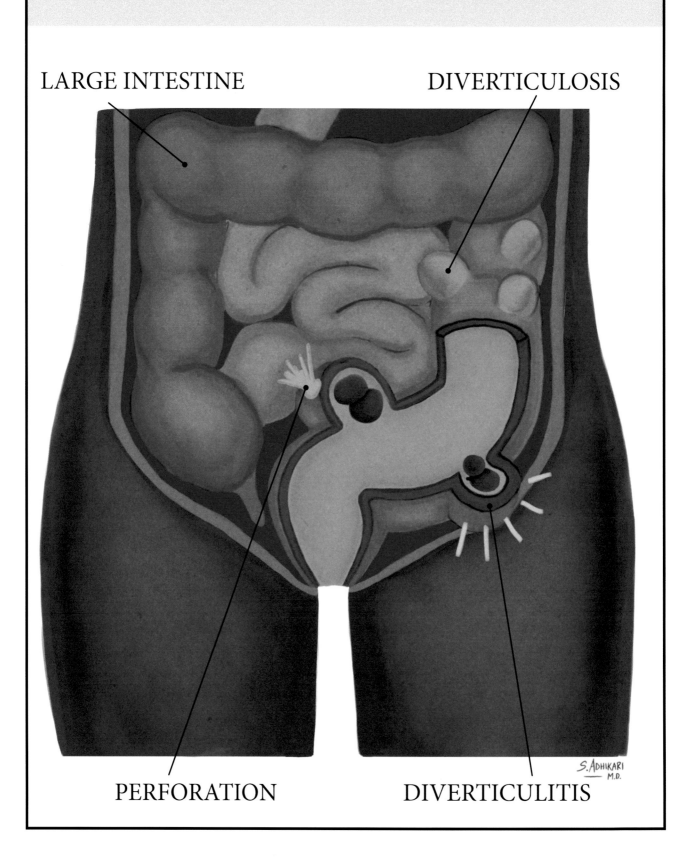

LARGE INTESTINE

DIVERTICULOSIS

PERFORATION

DIVERTICULITIS

CONSTIPATION

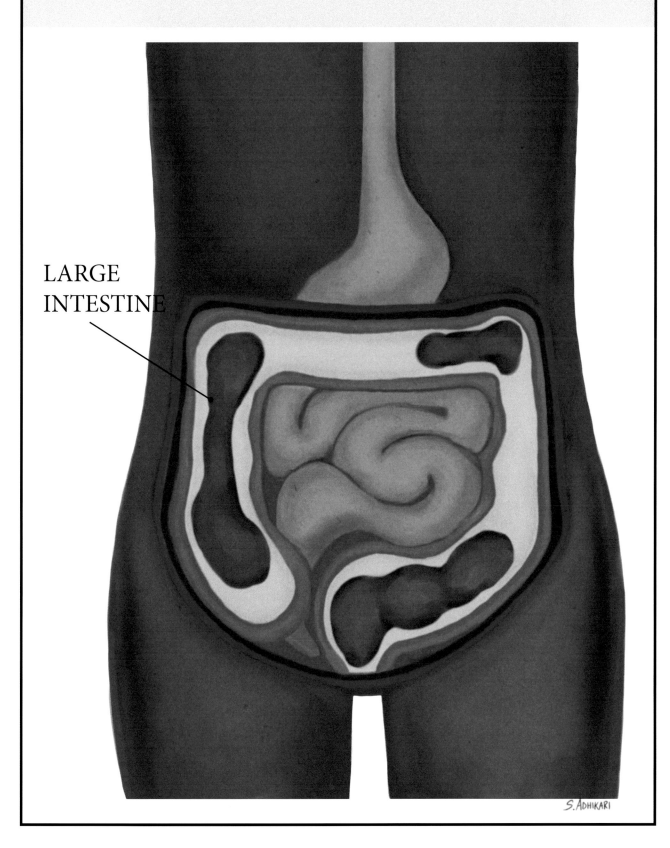

LARGE
INTESTINE

S.ADHIKARI

PERIRECTAL ABSCESS

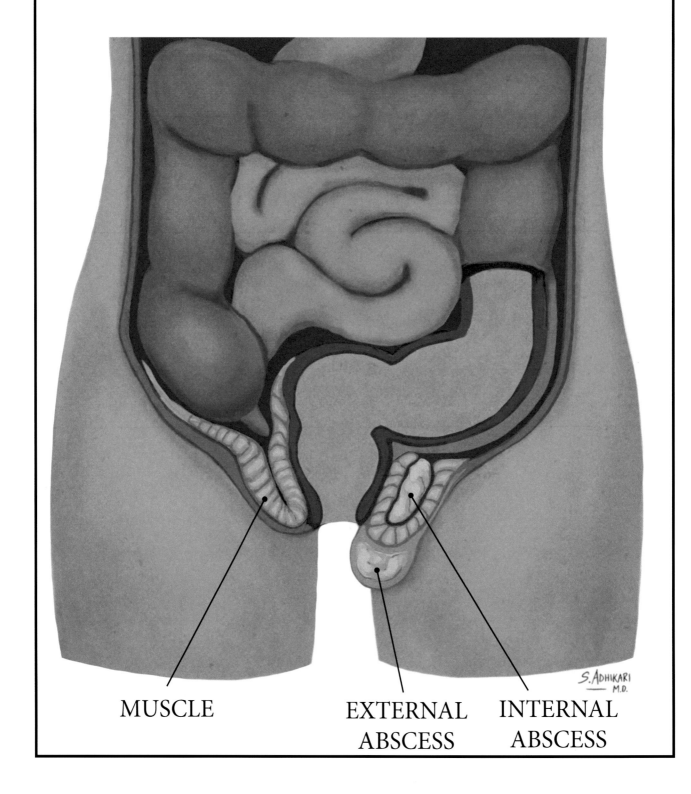

MUSCLE

EXTERNAL
ABSCESS

INTERNAL
ABSCESS

HEMORRHOIDS

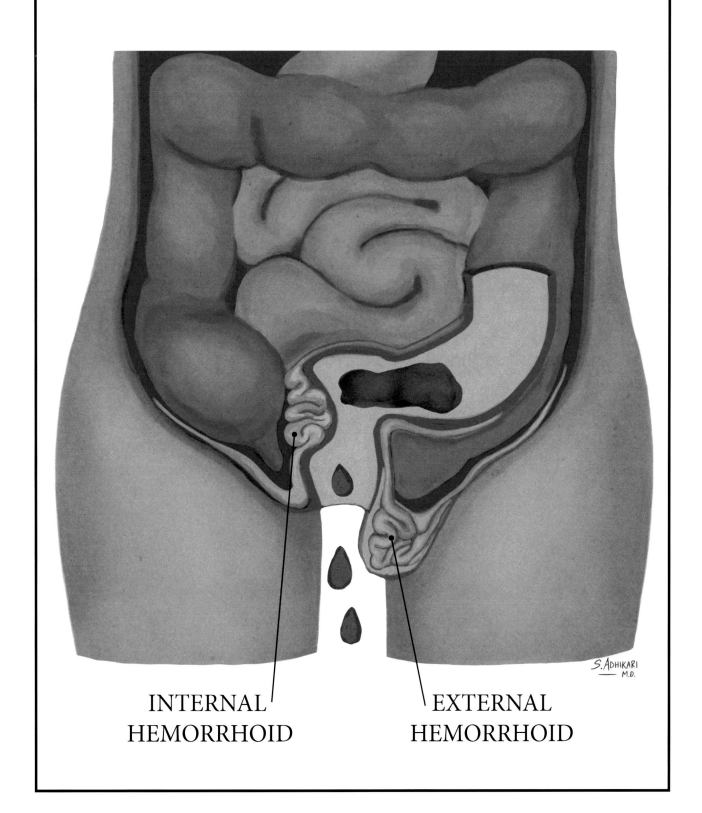

INTERNAL
HEMORRHOID

EXTERNAL
HEMORRHOID

APPENDICITIS

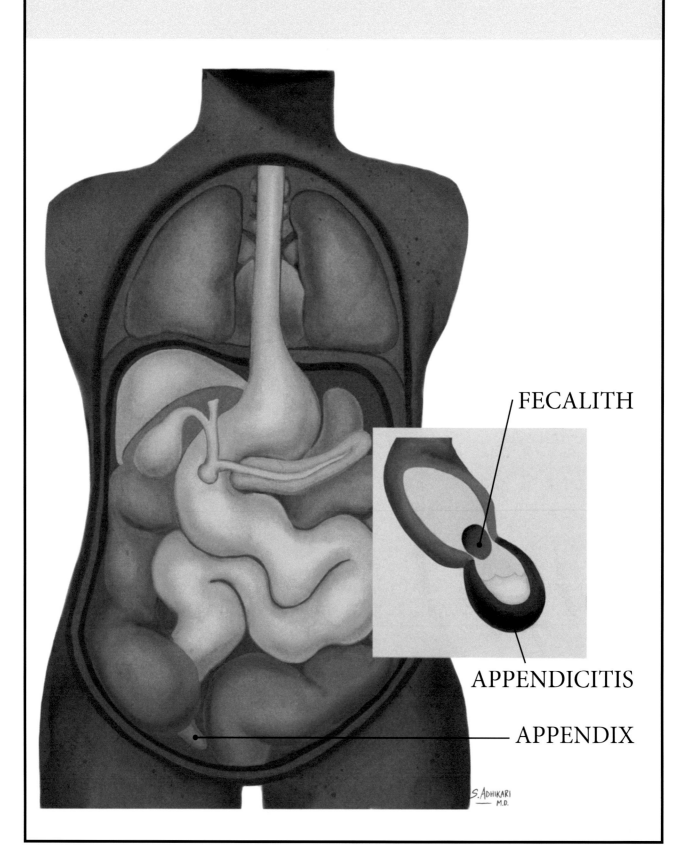

FECALITH

APPENDICITIS

APPENDIX

GENITOURINARY

KIDNEY STONE
NEPHROLITHIASIS

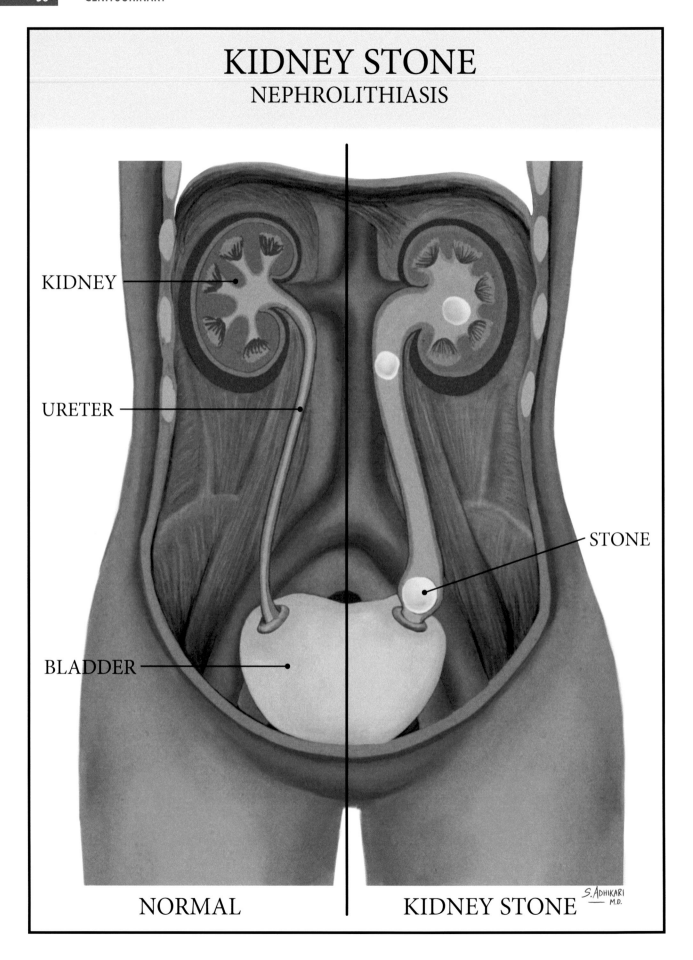

KIDNEY

URETER

STONE

BLADDER

NORMAL

KIDNEY STONE

URINARY TRACT INFECTION
CYSTITIS vs PYELONEPHRITIS

KIDNEY

BLADDER

BACTERIA

S. ADHIKARI
M.D.

ENLARGED PROSTATE
BENIGN PROSTATIC HYPERTROPHY (BPH)

KIDNEY

URETER

BLADDER

PROSTATE

URETHRA

S. ADHIKARI
M.D.

URINARY RETENTION

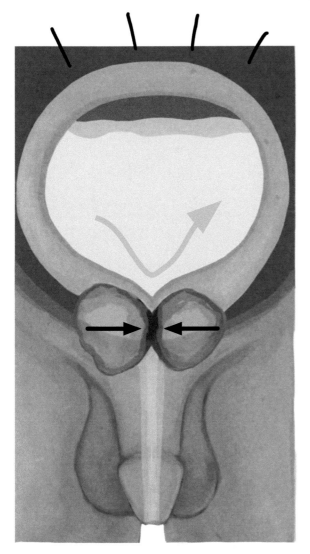

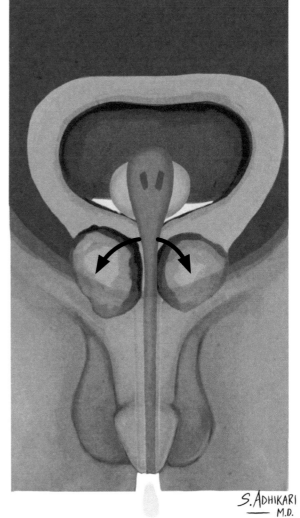

PROSTATE BLOCKS
URINE OUTFLOW

FOLEY CATHETER
PUSHES PROSTATE
ASIDE

TESTICULAR SWELLING
EPIDIDYMITIS

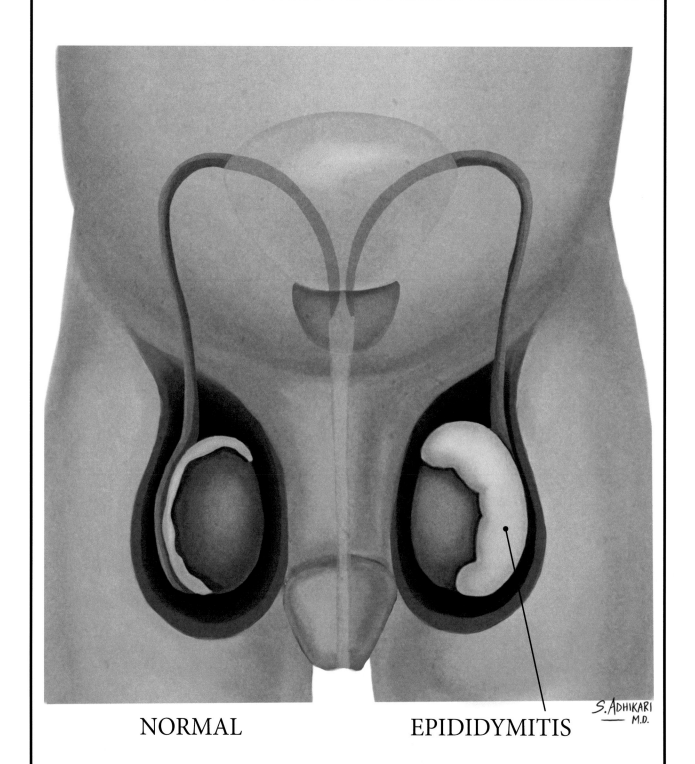

NORMAL   EPIDIDYMITIS

S. ADHIKARI
M.D.

TESTICULAR SWELLING
HYDROCELE vs VARICOCELE

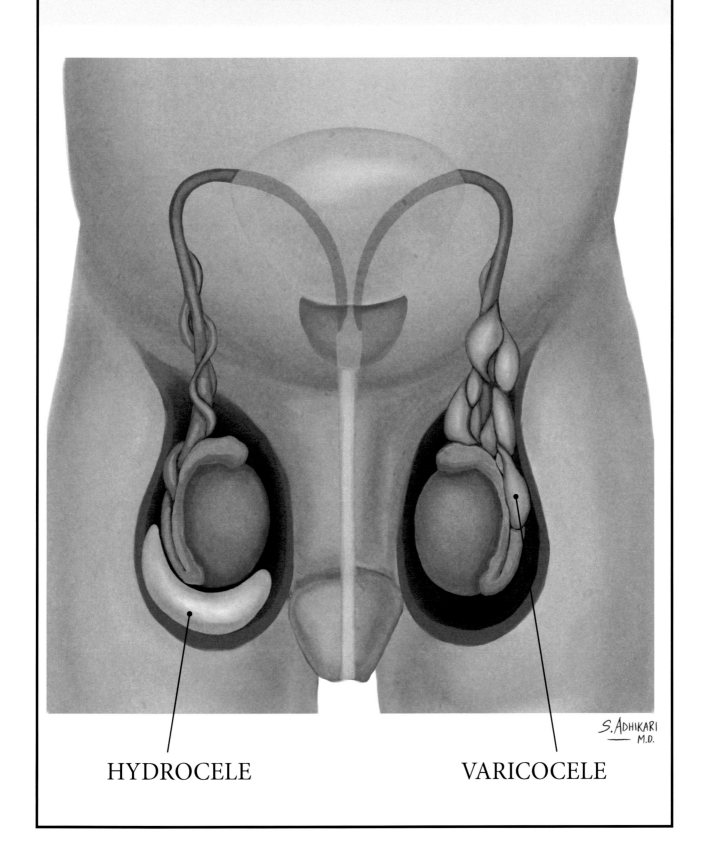

HYDROCELE   VARICOCELE

TESTICULAR TORSION

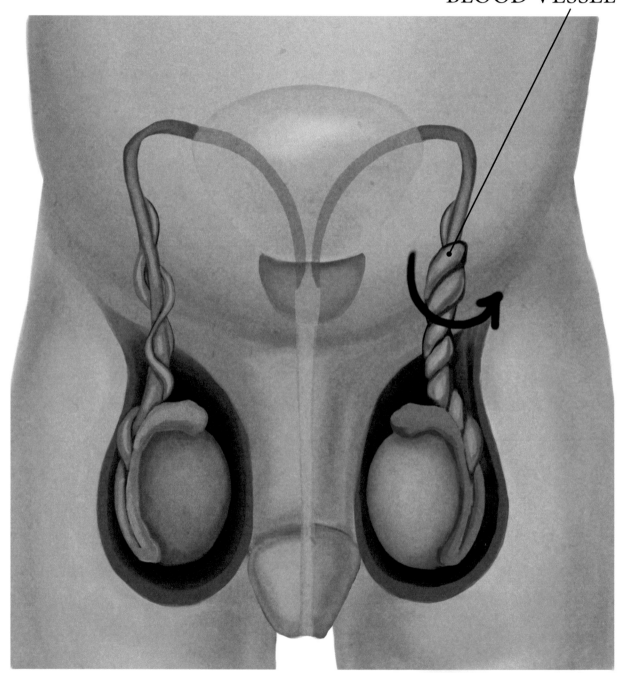

BLOOD VESSEL

S. ADHIKARI
M.D.

NORMAL   TORSION

OVARIAN TORSION

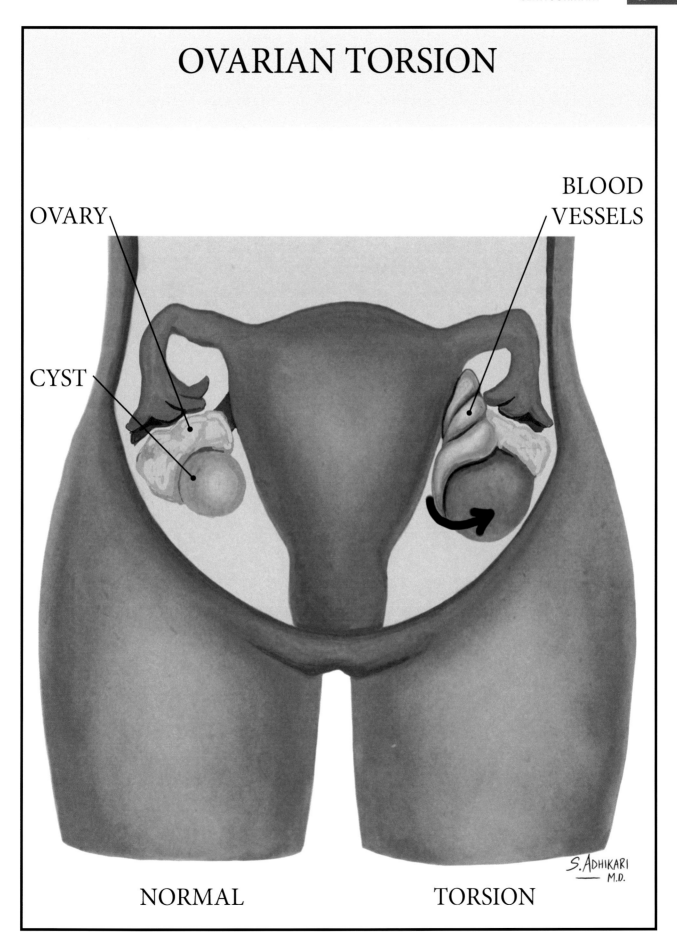

OVARY

CYST

BLOOD VESSELS

S. ADHIKARI M.D.

NORMAL   TORSION

OVARIAN CYST
NORMAL CYST vs RUPTURED CYST

OVARY

CYST

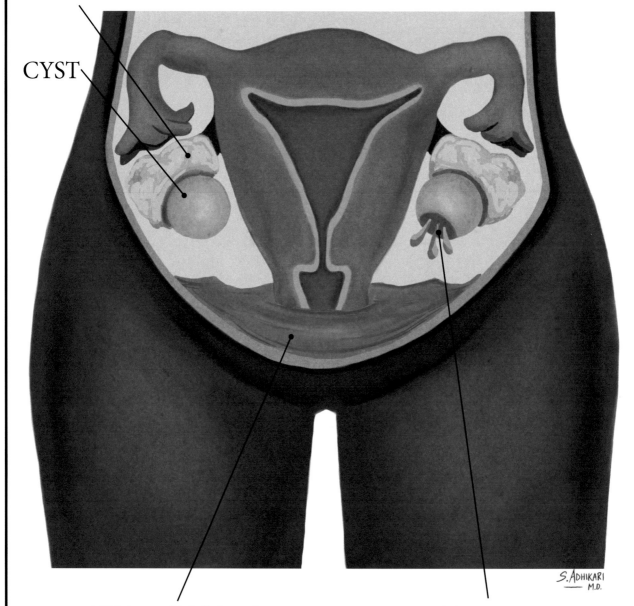

FLUID SETTLES
IN THE ABDOMINAL
CAVITY

RUPTURED
OVARIAN CYST

EARLY PREGNANCY
ABDOMINAL PAIN &/OR VAGINAL BLEEDING

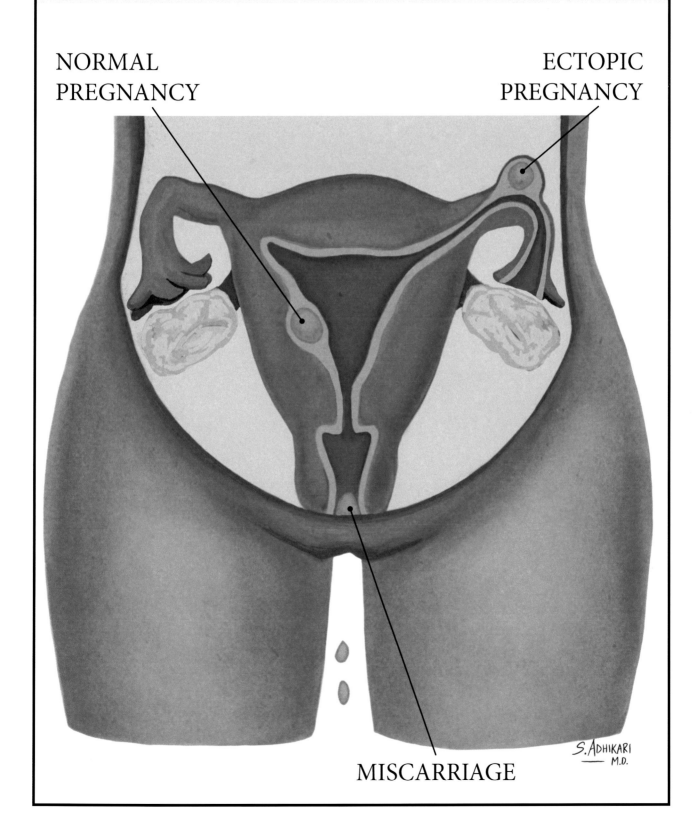

NORMAL
PREGNANCY

ECTOPIC
PREGNANCY

MISCARRIAGE

S. ADHIKARI
M.D.

FIBROIDS
LEIOMYOMA

UTERUS

FIBROIDS

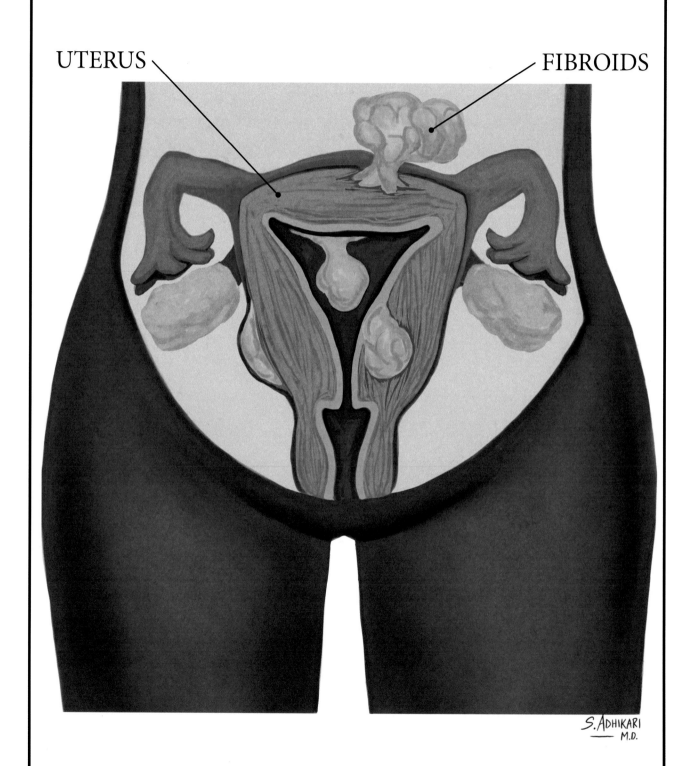

S. Adhikari
M.D.

IRREGULAR PERIODS
ABNORMAL UTERINE BLEEDING

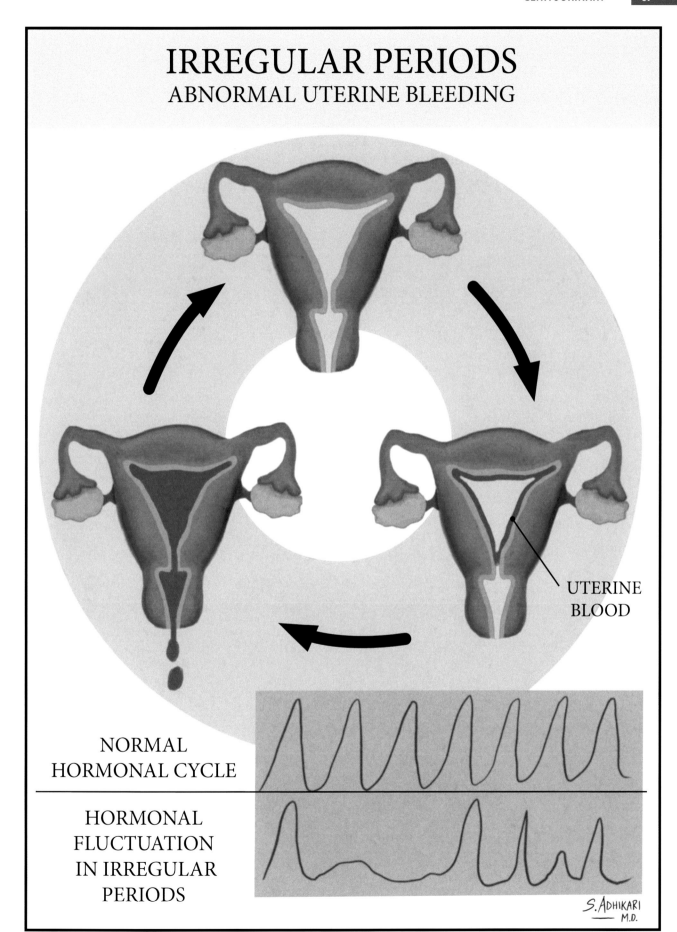

UTERINE BLOOD

NORMAL HORMONAL CYCLE

HORMONAL FLUCTUATION IN IRREGULAR PERIODS

S. ADHIKARI M.D.

YEAST INFECTION
VAGINAL CANDIDIASIS

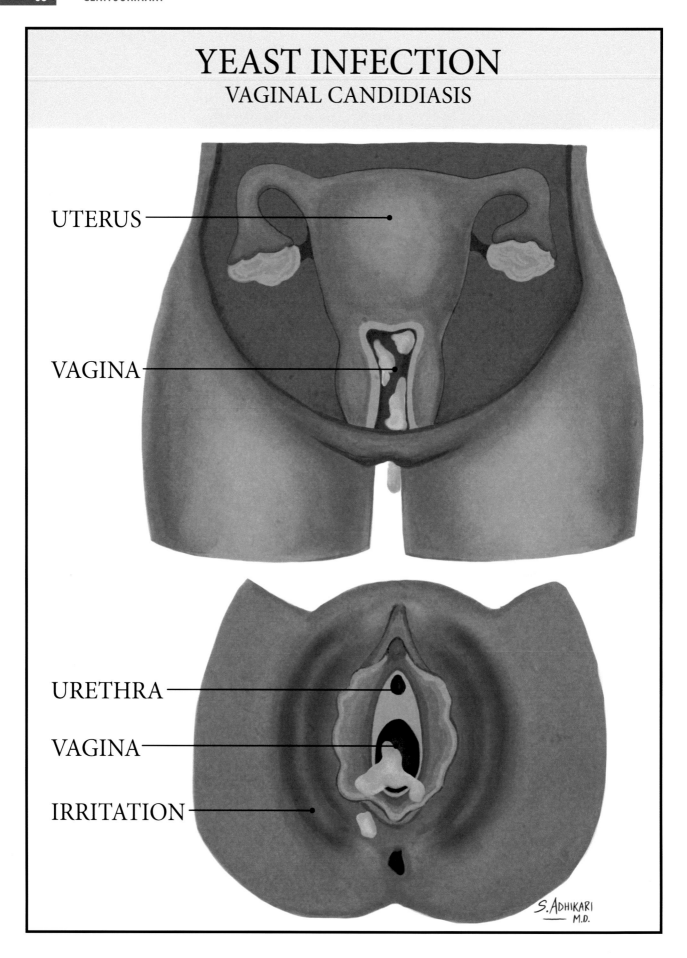

UTERUS

VAGINA

URETHRA

VAGINA

IRRITATION

S. ADHIKARI
M.D.

VAGINAL DISCHARGE
BACTERIAL VAGINOSIS

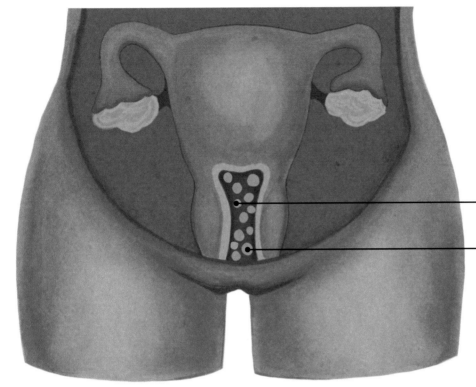

GOOD
BACTERIA

BAD
BACTERIA

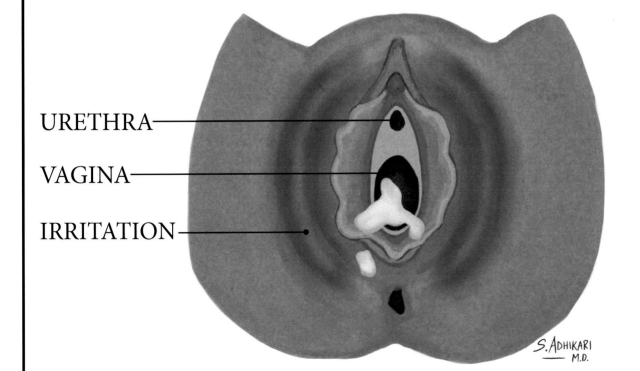

URETHRA

VAGINA

IRRITATION

S. ADHIKARI
M.D.

PELVIC INFECTION
PELVIC INFLAMMATORY DISEASE (PID) &
TUBO-OVARIAN ABSCESS (TOA)

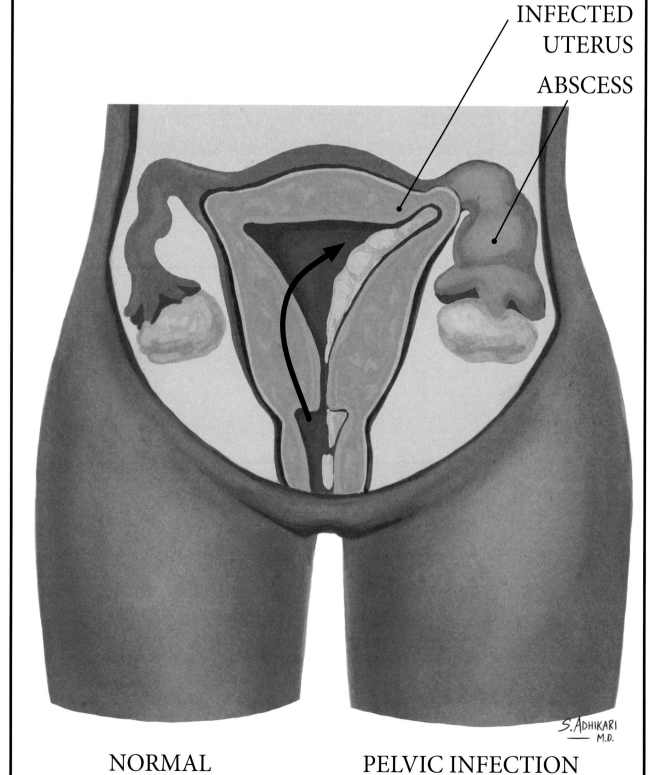

INFECTED UTERUS

ABSCESS

S. Adhikari
M.D.

NORMAL   PELVIC INFECTION

SEXUALLY TRANSMITTED INFECTION

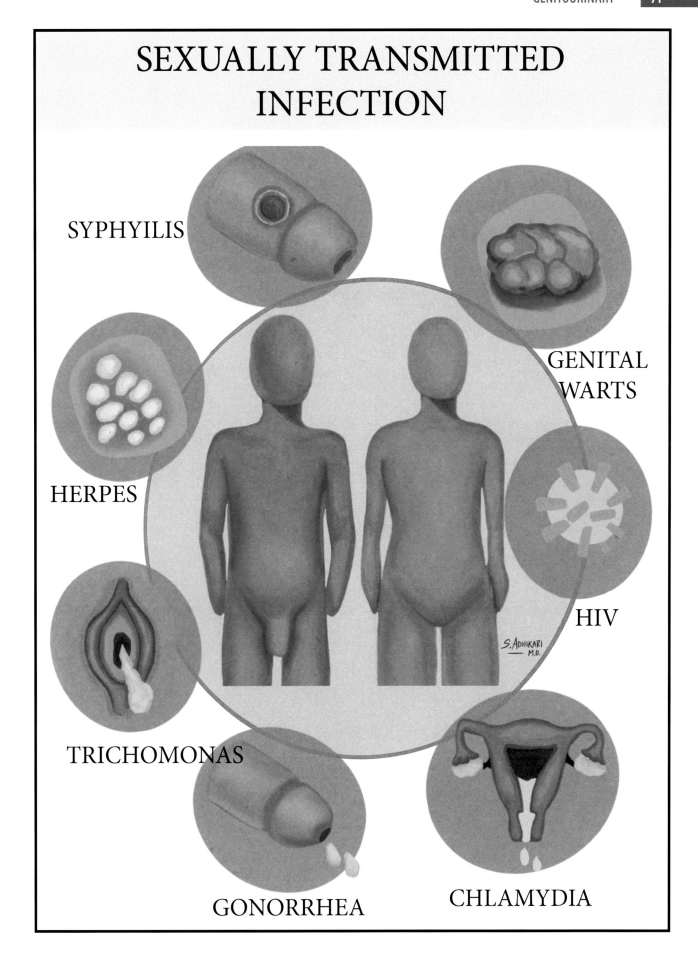

SYPHYILIS

GENITAL WARTS

HERPES

HIV

TRICHOMONAS

GONORRHEA

CHLAMYDIA

S. ADHIKARI M.D.

LOWER ABDOMEN
MALE vs FEMALE

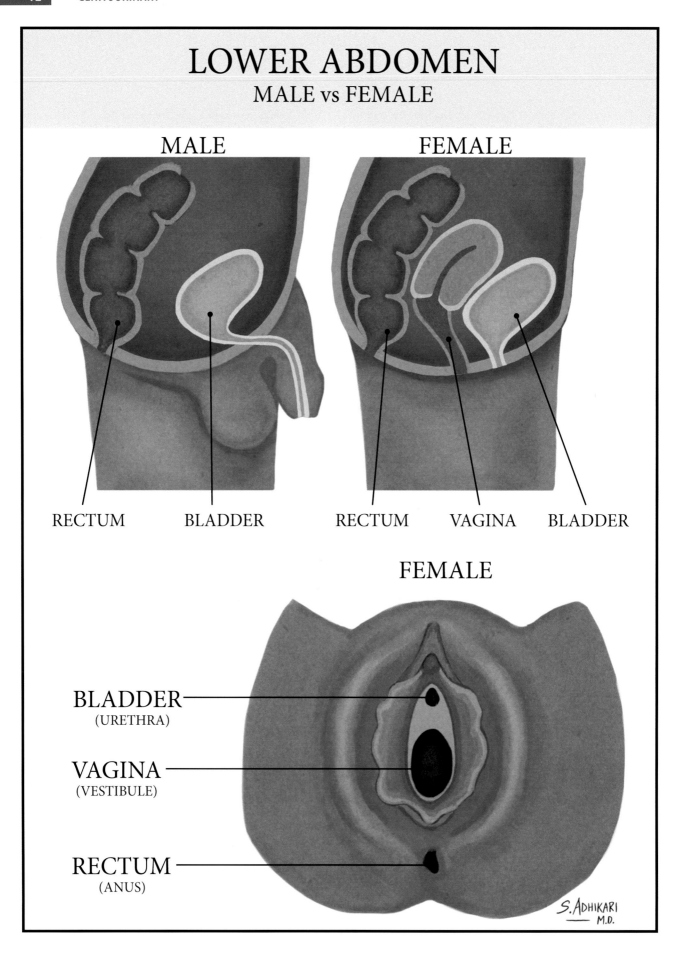

MALE

FEMALE

RECTUM   BLADDER   RECTUM   VAGINA   BLADDER

FEMALE

BLADDER
(URETHRA)

VAGINA
(VESTIBULE)

RECTUM
(ANUS)

S. ADHIKARI
M.D.

ORTHOPEDICS

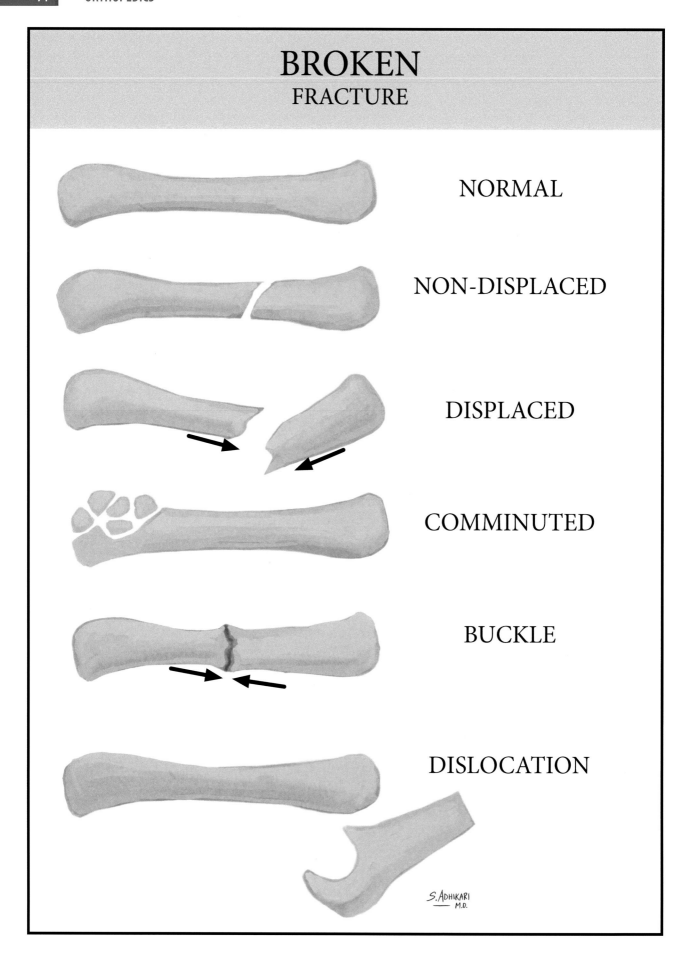

BROKEN
FRACTURE

NORMAL

NON-DISPLACED

DISPLACED

COMMINUTED

BUCKLE

DISLOCATION

S. Adhikari
M.D.

GROWTH PLATE INJURY

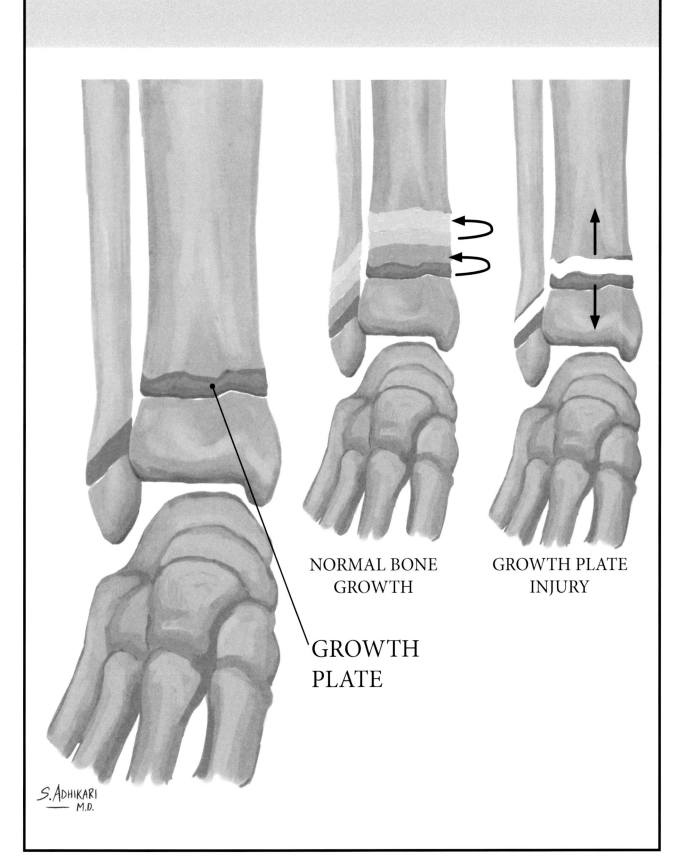

GROWTH
PLATE

NORMAL BONE
GROWTH

GROWTH PLATE
INJURY

S.ADHIKARI
M.D.

ARTHRITIS
DEGENERATIVE JOINT DISEASE

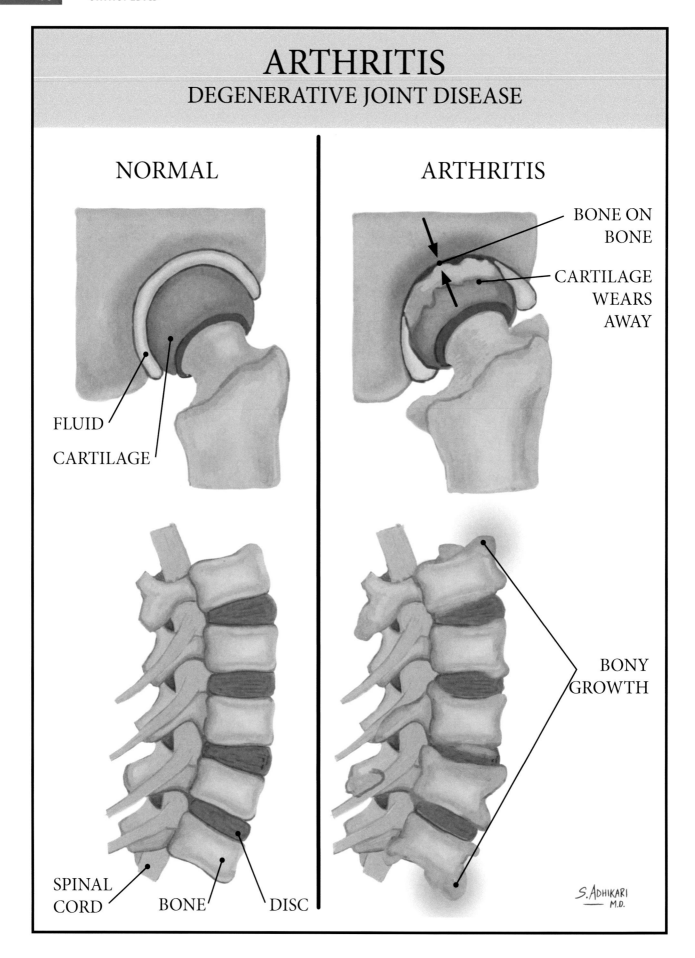

NORMAL

ARTHRITIS

BONE ON
BONE

CARTILAGE
WEARS
AWAY

FLUID

CARTILAGE

BONY
GROWTH

SPINAL
CORD   BONE   DISC

S. ADHIKARI
M.D.

BURSITIS

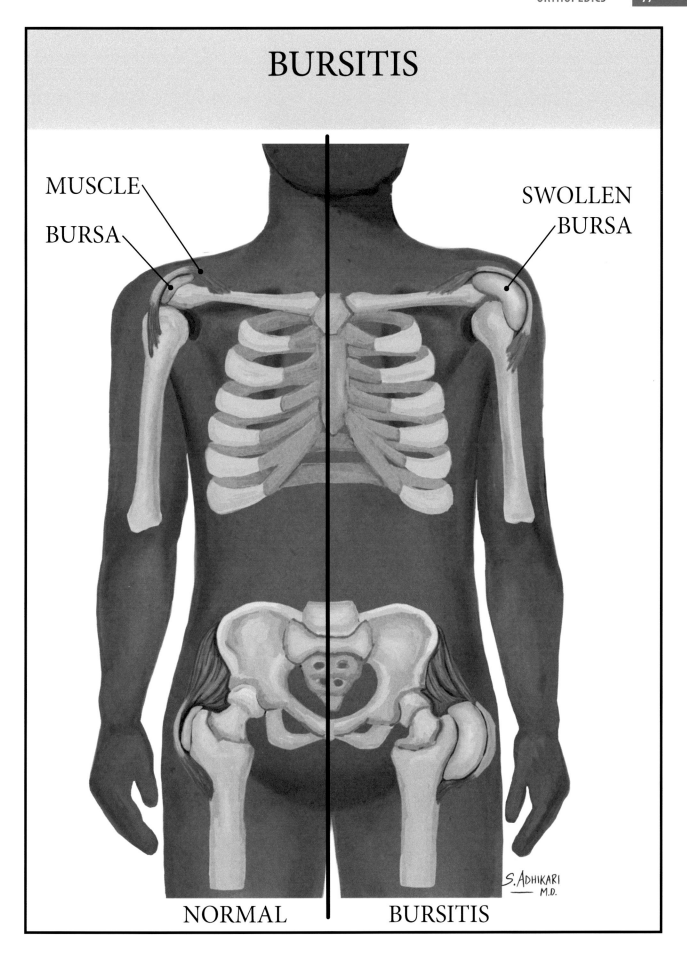

MUSCLE

BURSA

SWOLLEN
BURSA

S. ADHIKARI
M.D.

NORMAL   BURSITIS

RIB FRACTURE

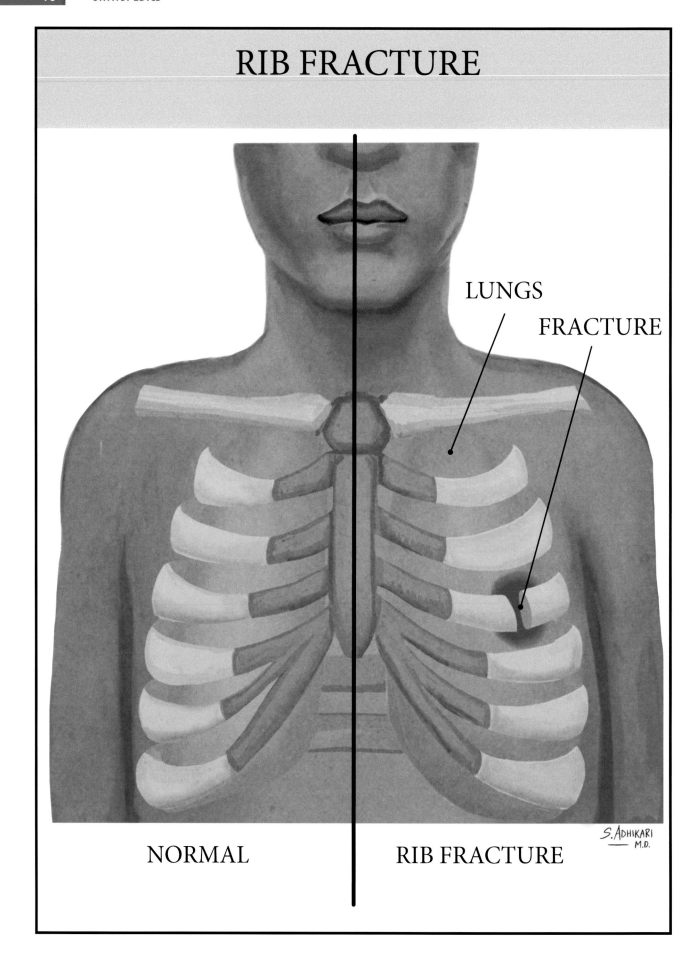

LUNGS

FRACTURE

S. ADHIKARI
M.D.

NORMAL   RIB FRACTURE

COLLAPSED LUNG
PNEUMOTHORAX

LUNGS

LAYERS

RIBS

COLLAPSED LUNG

AIR

CHEST TUBE

S. ADHIKARI
M.D.

NORMAL

COLLAPSED LUNG

BACK PAIN
MUSCULOSKELETAL

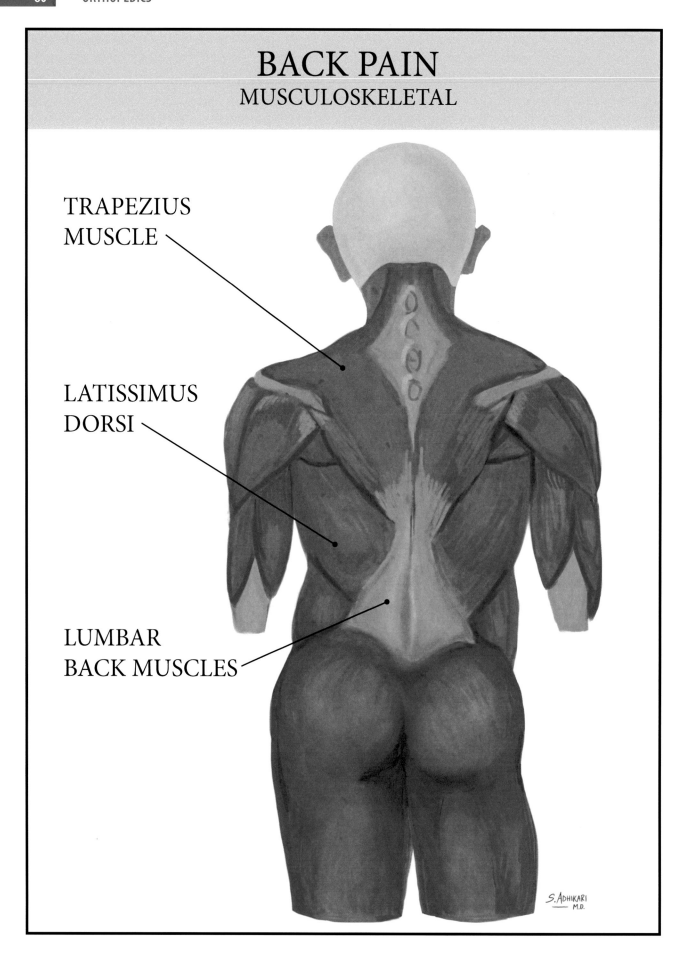

TRAPEZIUS
MUSCLE

LATISSIMUS
DORSI

LUMBAR
BACK MUSCLES

S. ADHIKARI
M.D.

BACK PAIN
SACROILIITIS

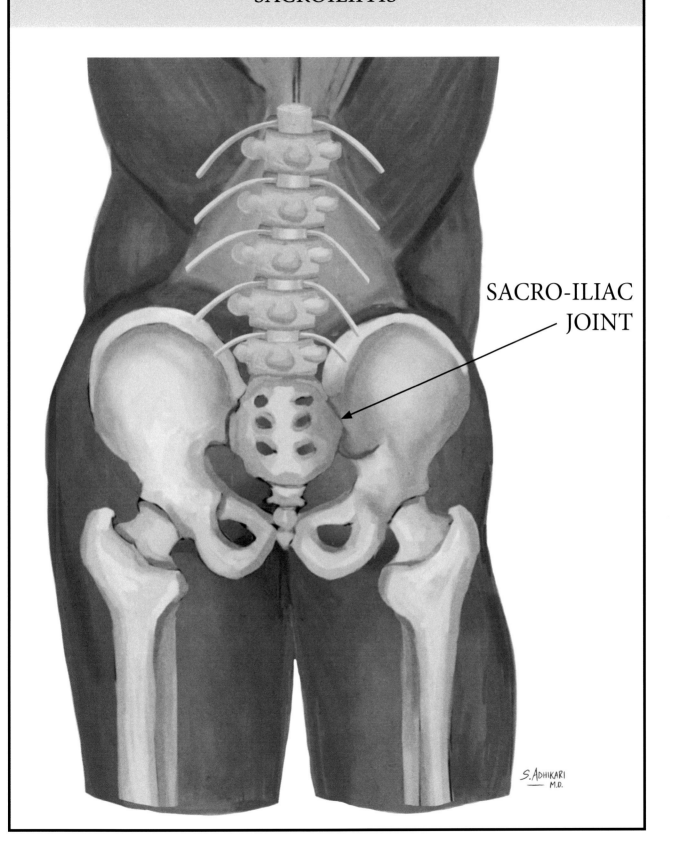

SACRO-ILIAC
JOINT

S. ADHIKARI
M.D.

BACK PAIN
SIDE VIEW

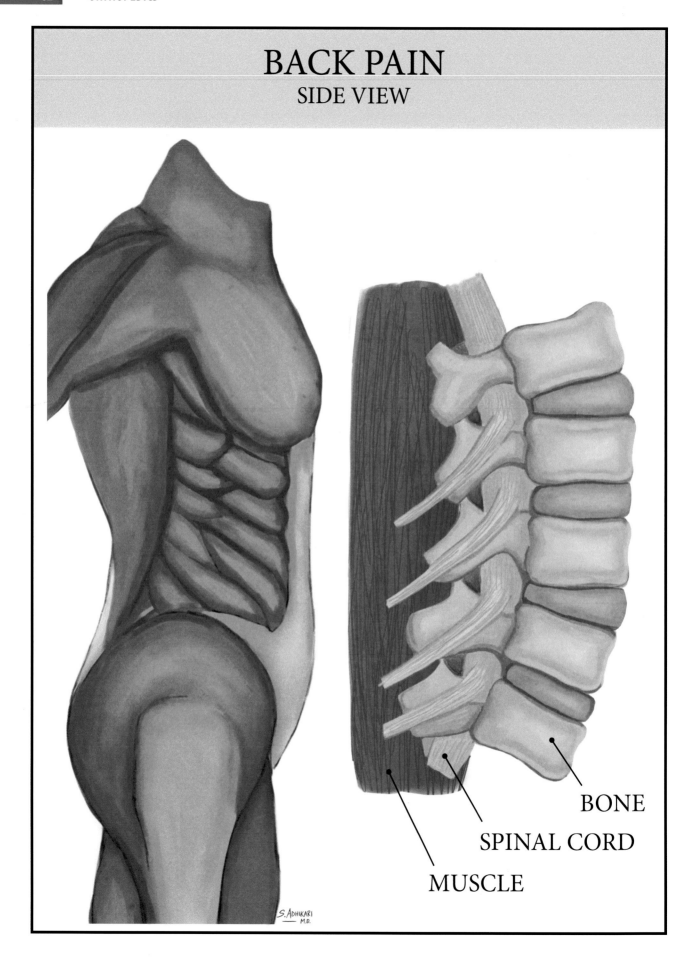

BONE

SPINAL CORD

MUSCLE

S. ADHIKARI
M.D.

SCIATICA
LUMBAR RADICULOPATHY

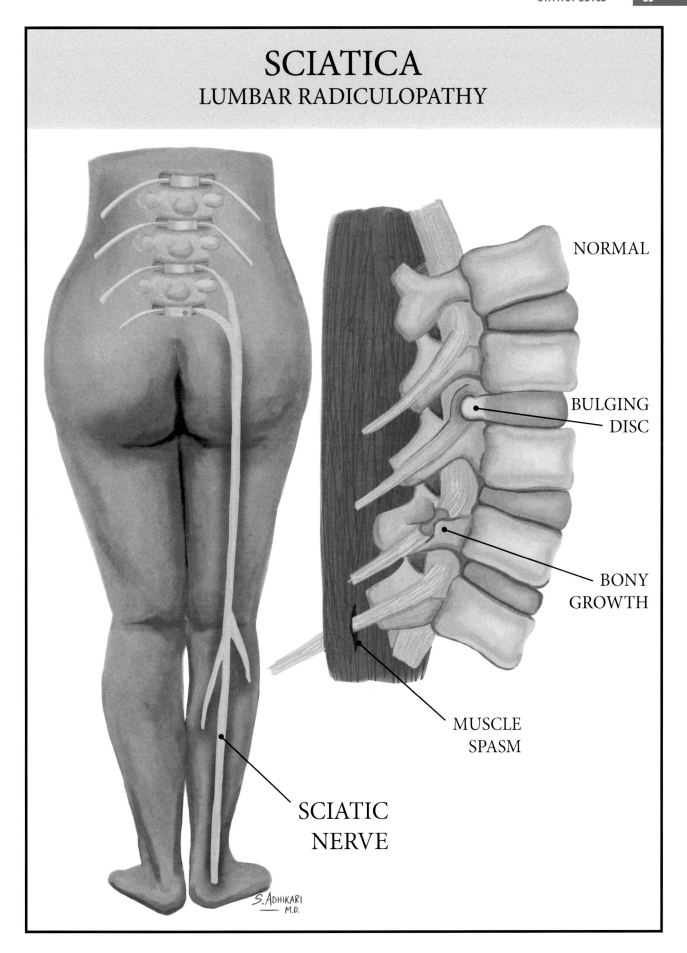

NORMAL

BULGING
DISC

BONY
GROWTH

MUSCLE
SPASM

SCIATIC
NERVE

S. ADHIKARI
M.D.

NECK PAIN
CERVICAL STRAIN

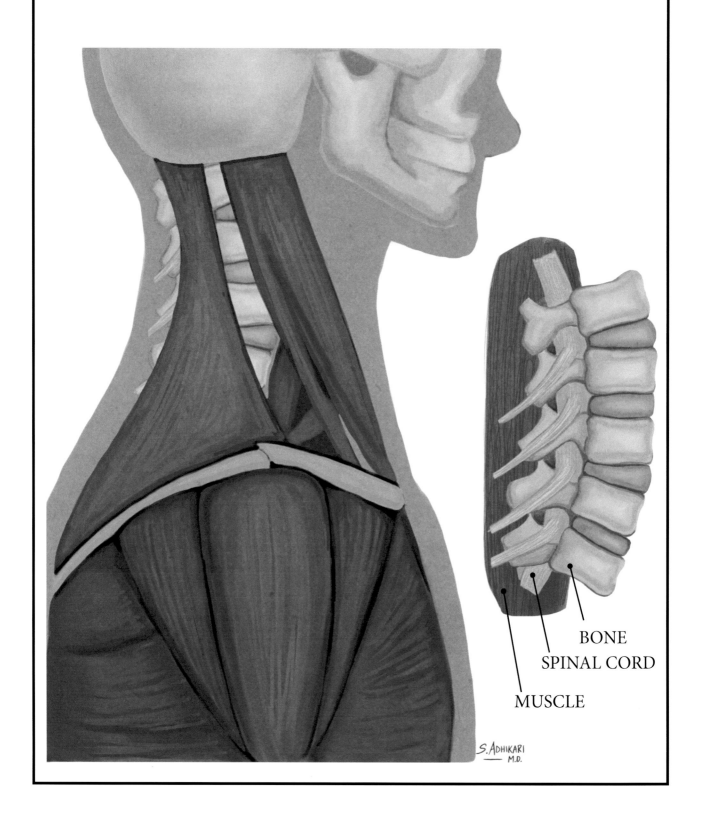

BONE

SPINAL CORD

MUSCLE

S. ADHIKARI
M.D.

NECK & BACK STRAIN
MOTOR VEHICLE ACCIDENT (MVA)

TRAPEZIUS
MUSCLE

LUMBAR
MUSCLE

S. ADHIKARI
M.D.

KNEE ARTHRITIS
OSTEOARTHRITIS

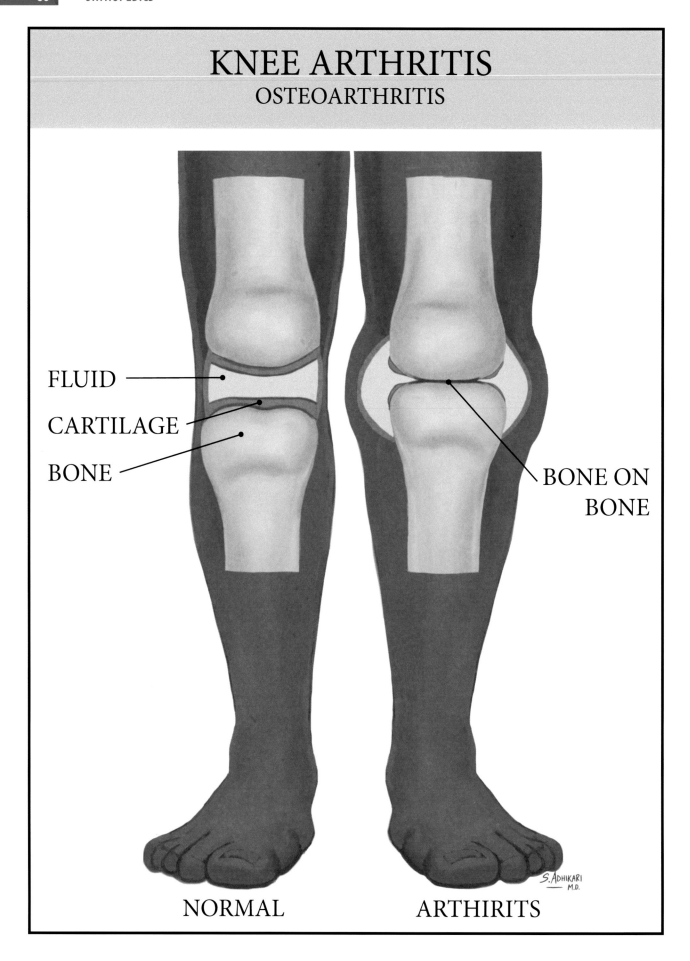

FLUID

CARTILAGE

BONE

BONE ON
BONE

S. Adhikari
M.D.

NORMAL   ARTHIRITS

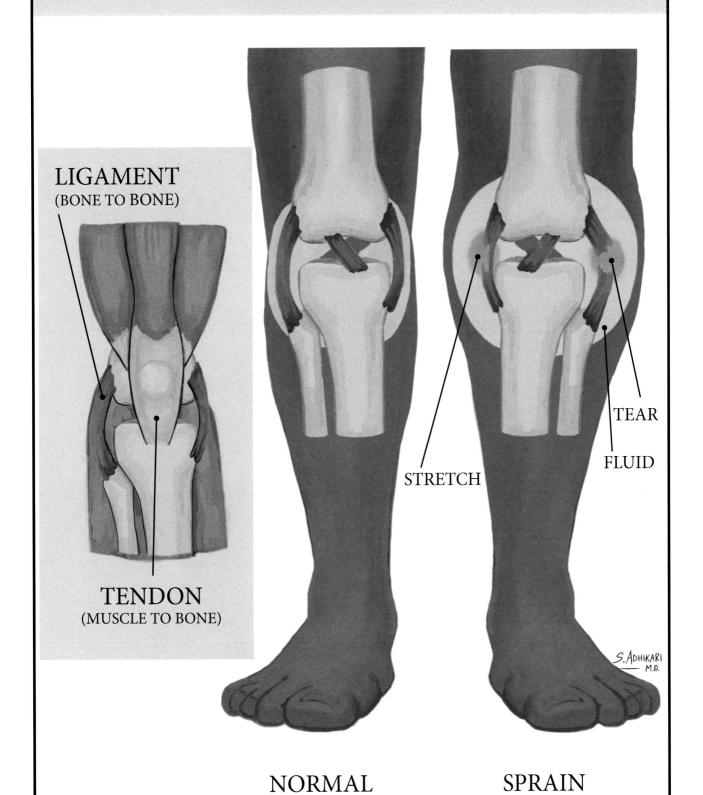

KNEE PAIN
FRACTURE vs SPRAIN

LIGAMENT
(BONE TO BONE)

TENDON
(MUSCLE TO BONE)

STRETCH

TEAR

FLUID

S. ADHIKARI
M.D.

NORMAL

SPRAIN

JOINT DISEASE
NORMAL ANATOMY

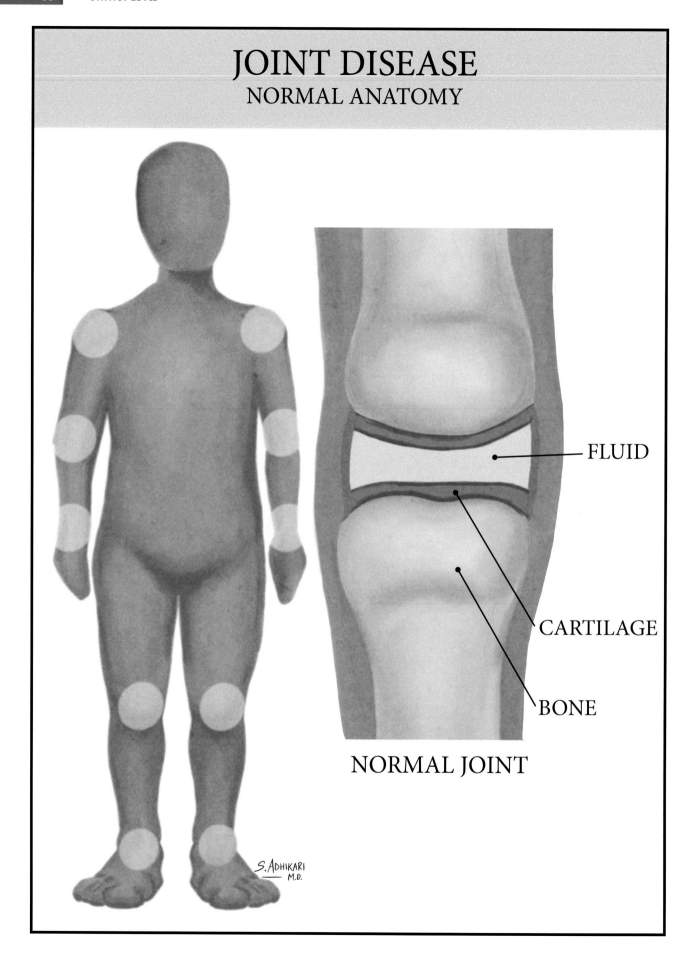

FLUID

CARTILAGE

BONE

NORMAL JOINT

INFLAMED JOINT
GOUT vs SEPTIC JOINT

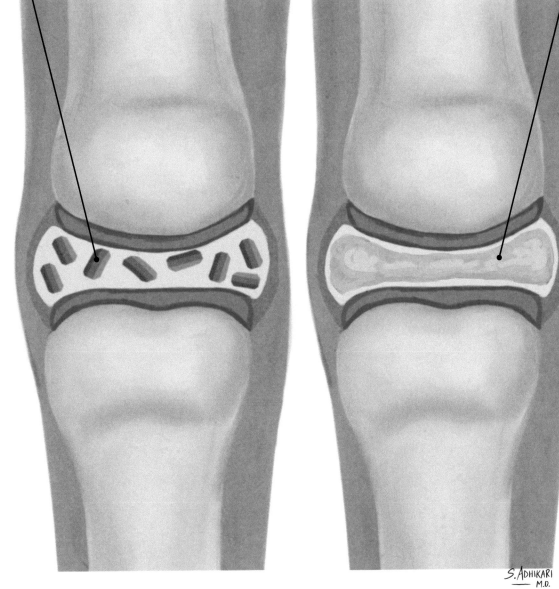

CRYSTALS

PUS

GOUT

SEPTIC JOINT

S. ADHIKARI
M.D.

BAKER'S CYST

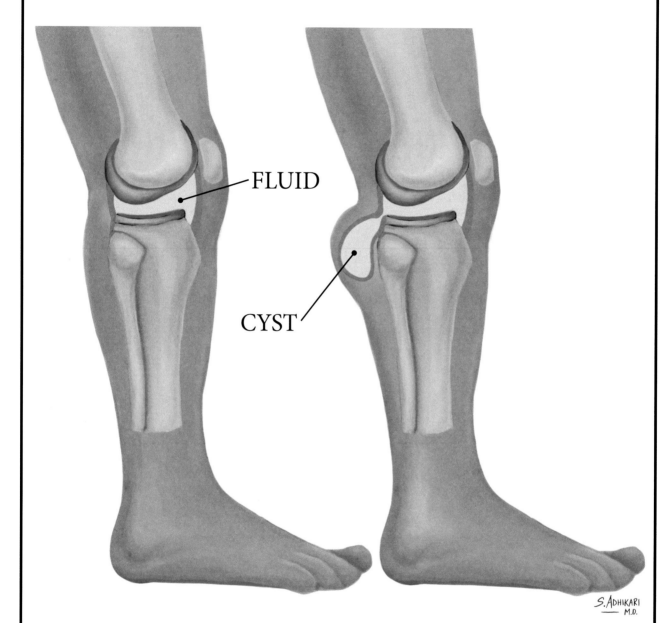

NORMAL

BAKER'S CYST

ANKLE PAIN
FRACTURE vs SPRAIN

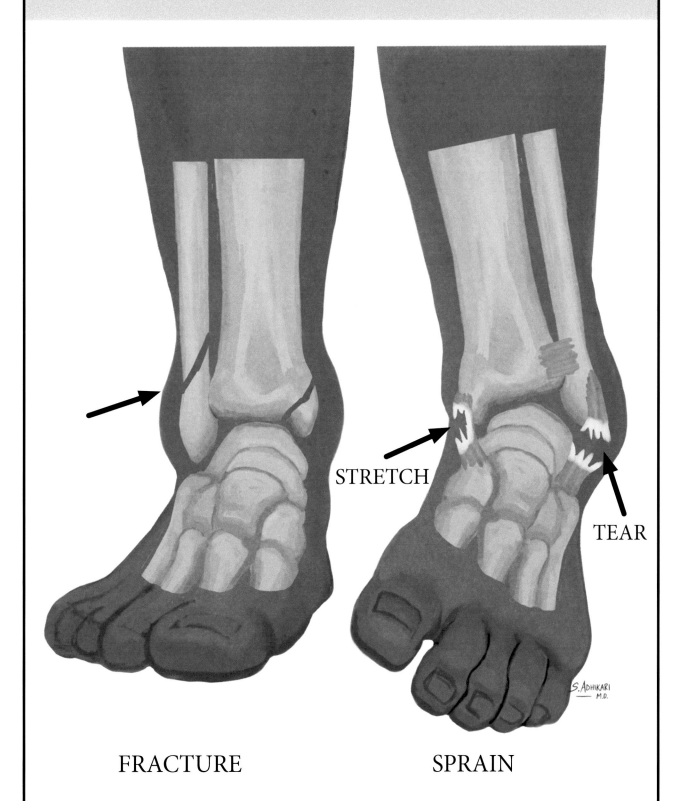

STRETCH

TEAR

FRACTURE

SPRAIN

S. ADHIKARI
M.D.

WRIST PAIN
CARPAL TUNNEL SYNDROME

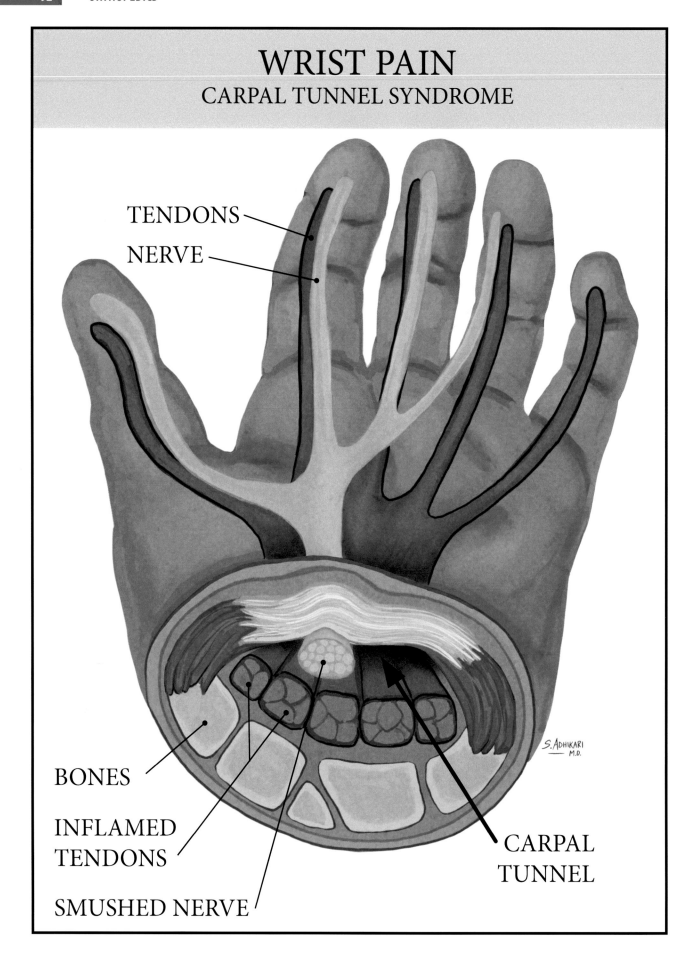

TENDONS

NERVE

BONES

INFLAMED
TENDONS

SMUSHED NERVE

CARPAL
TUNNEL

S. ADHIKARI
M.D.

FOOT PAIN
PLANTAR FASCIITIS

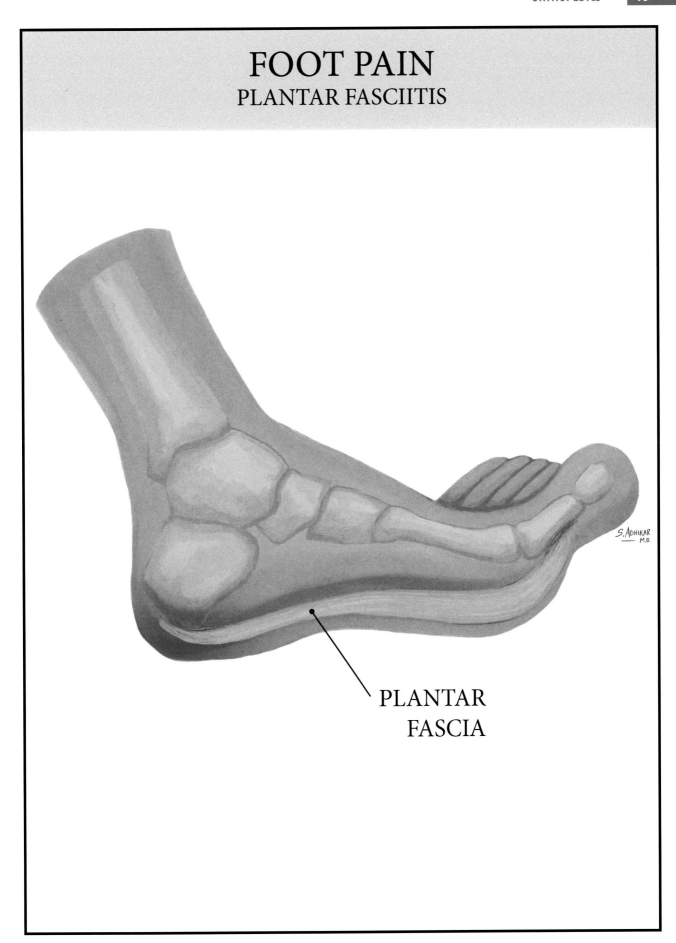

PLANTAR
FASCIA

BROKEN BACK
COMPRESSION FRACTURE

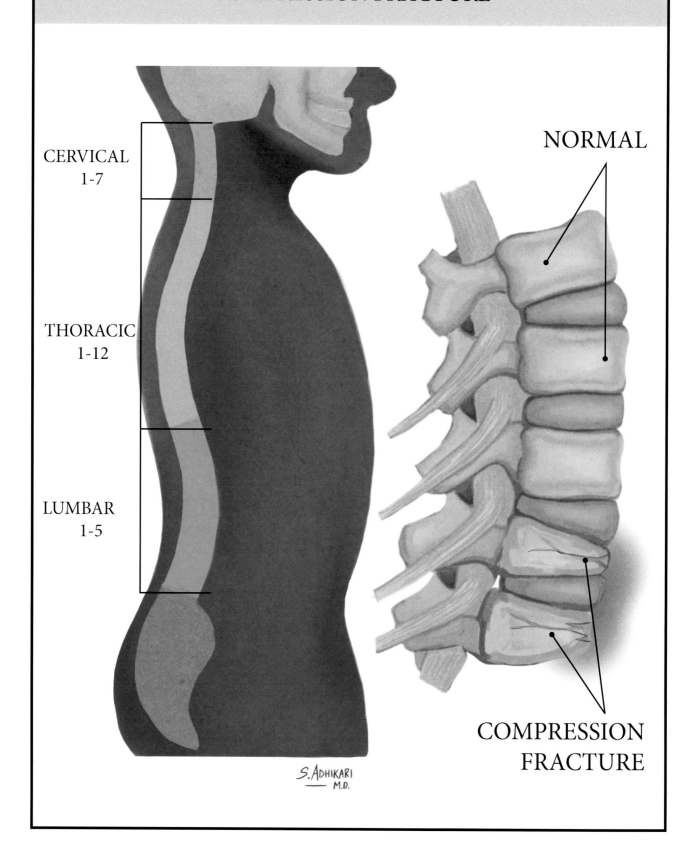

CERVICAL
1-7

THORACIC
1-12

LUMBAR
1-5

NORMAL

COMPRESSION
FRACTURE

S. ADHIKARI
M.D.

NEUROLOGY

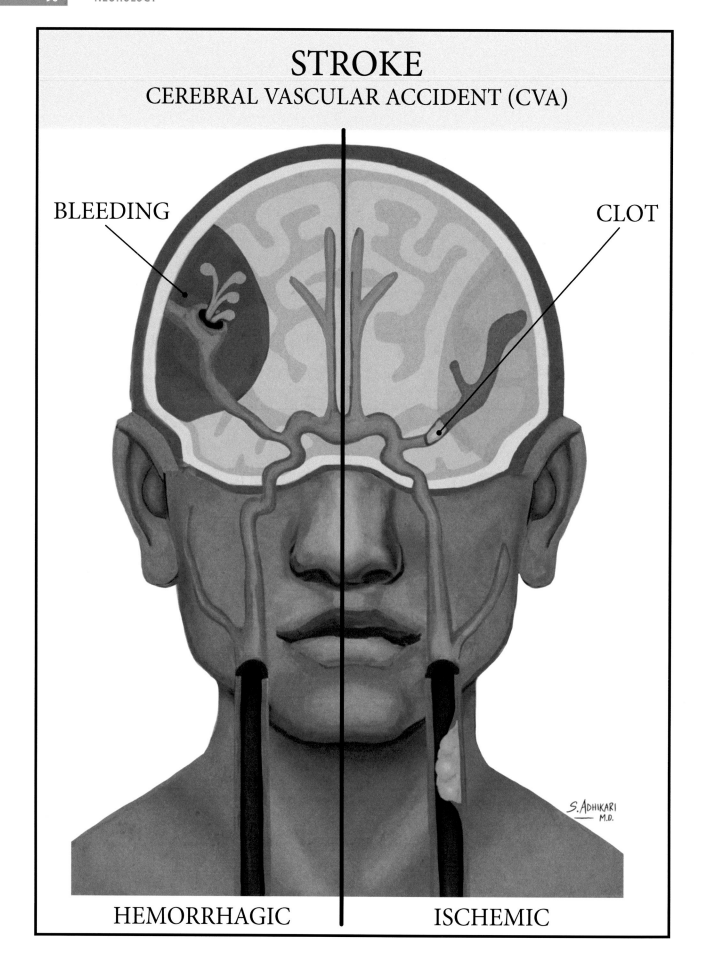

STROKE
CEREBRAL VASCULAR ACCIDENT (CVA)

BLEEDING

CLOT

HEMORRHAGIC

ISCHEMIC

S. ADHIKARI
M.D.

MINI-STROKE
TRANSIENT ISCHEMIC ATTACK (TIA)

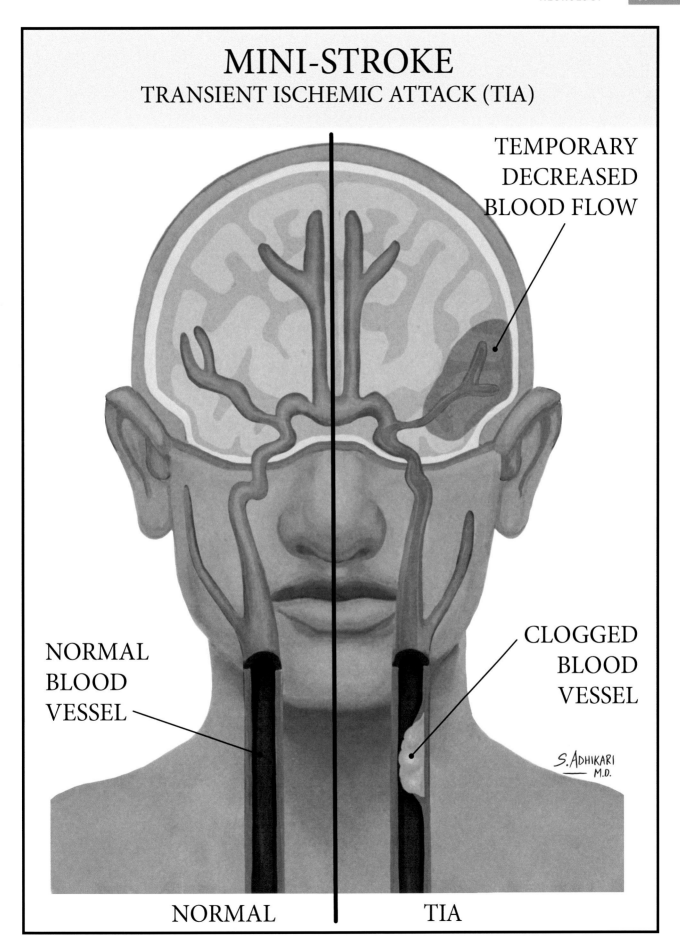

TEMPORARY
DECREASED
BLOOD FLOW

CLOGGED
BLOOD
VESSEL

NORMAL
BLOOD
VESSEL

S. ADHIKARI
M.D.

NORMAL   TIA

BRAIN BLEED
INTRACRANIAL HEMORRHAGE (ICH)

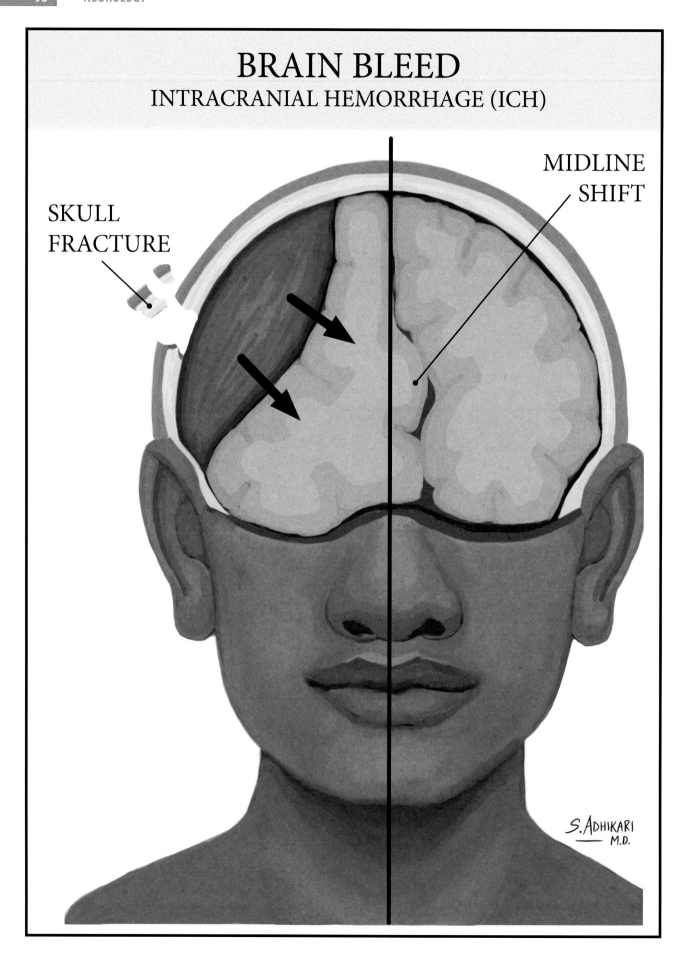

MIDLINE
SHIFT

SKULL
FRACTURE

S.ADHIKARI
M.D.

BRAIN ANEURYSM
SUBARACHNOID HEMORRHAGE (SAH)

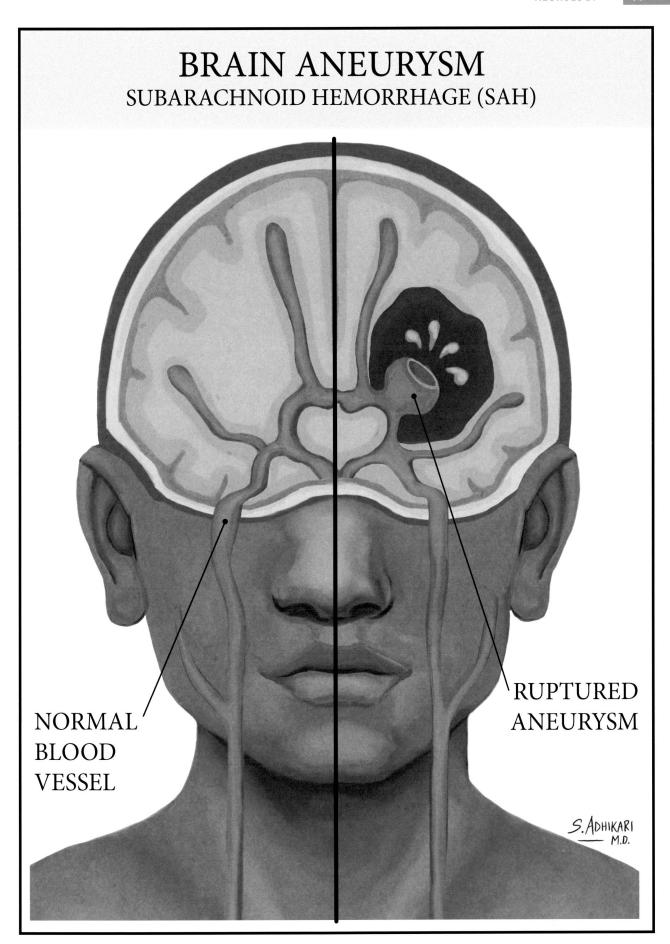

NORMAL
BLOOD
VESSEL

RUPTURED
ANEURYSM

S. ADHIKARI
M.D.

MENINGITIS

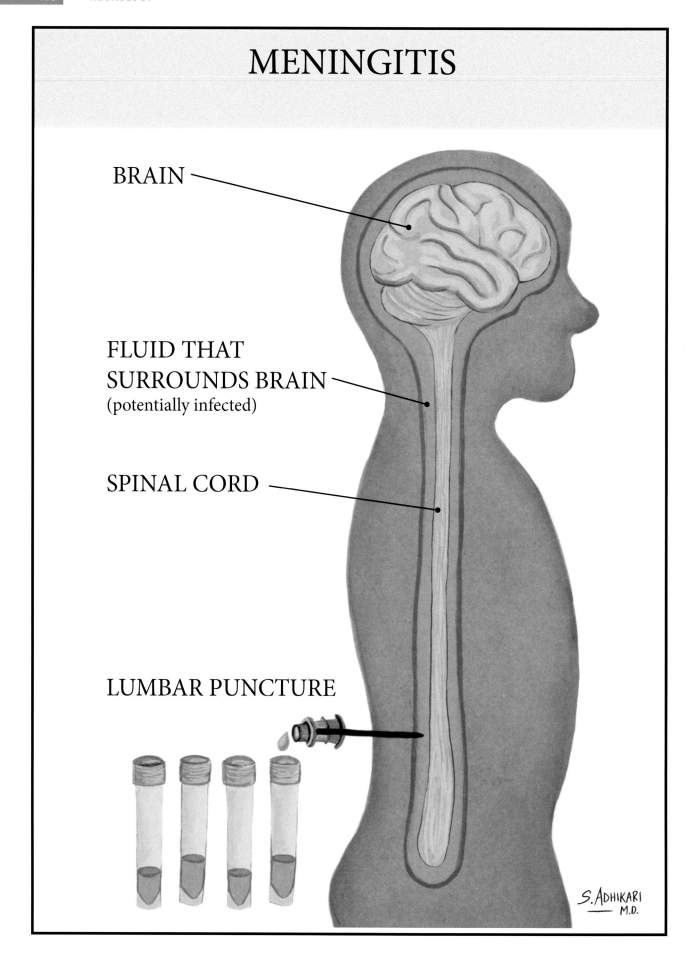

BRAIN

FLUID THAT
SURROUNDS BRAIN
(potentially infected)

SPINAL CORD

LUMBAR PUNCTURE

S. ADHIKARI
M.D.

DIZZINESS
BENIGN POSITIONAL VERTIGO (BPV)

NORMAL FLOW   BUMPY FLOW   NERVE

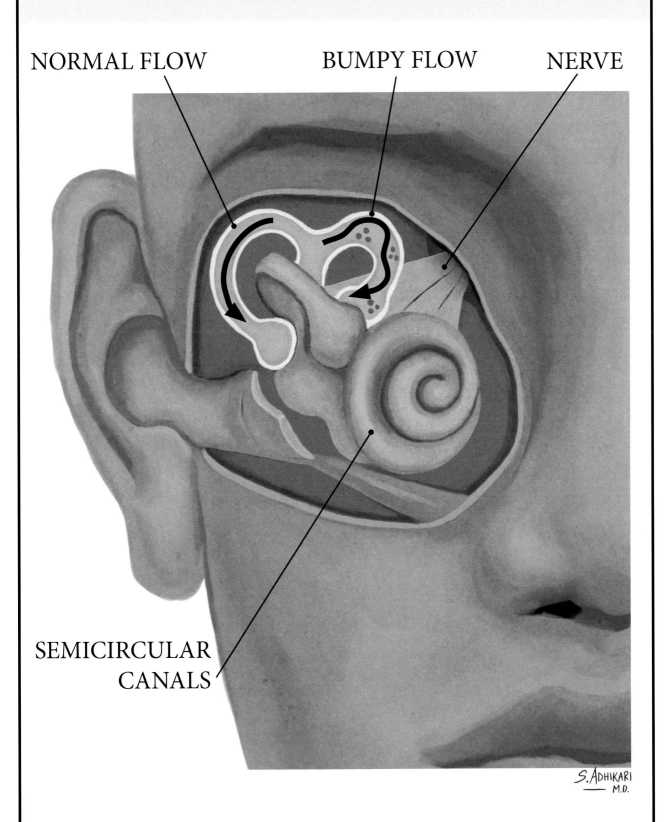

SEMICIRCULAR
CANALS

S. ADHIKARI
— M.D.

BELL'S PALSY
7th CRANIAL NERVE PALSY

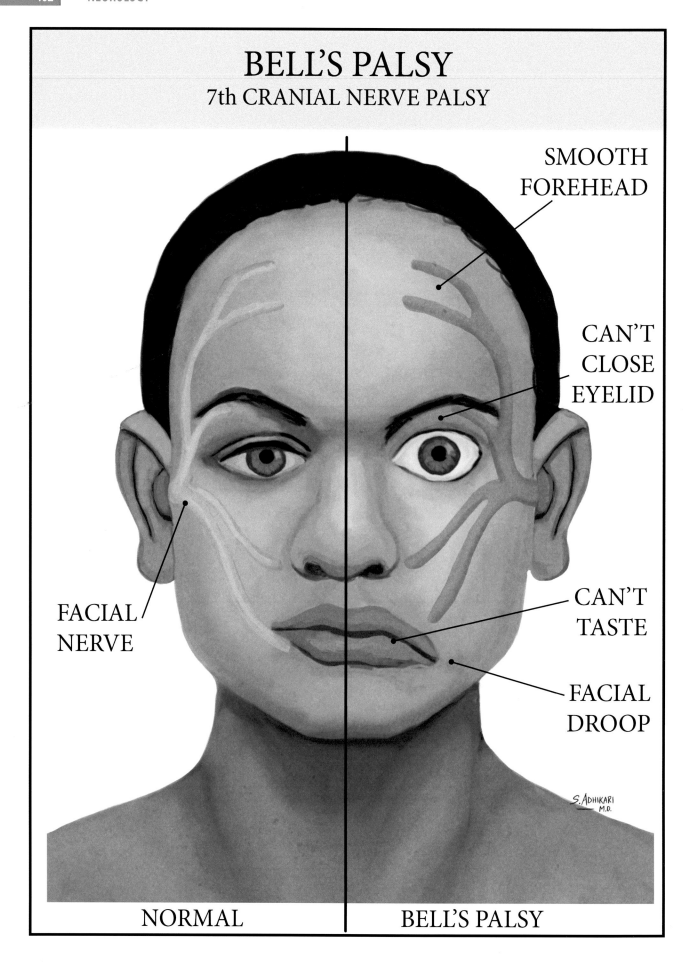

SMOOTH
FOREHEAD

CAN'T
CLOSE
EYELID

FACIAL
NERVE

CAN'T
TASTE

FACIAL
DROOP

NORMAL   BELL'S PALSY

CONCUSSION
CLOSED HEAD INJURY

BRAIN SITS
IN FLUID

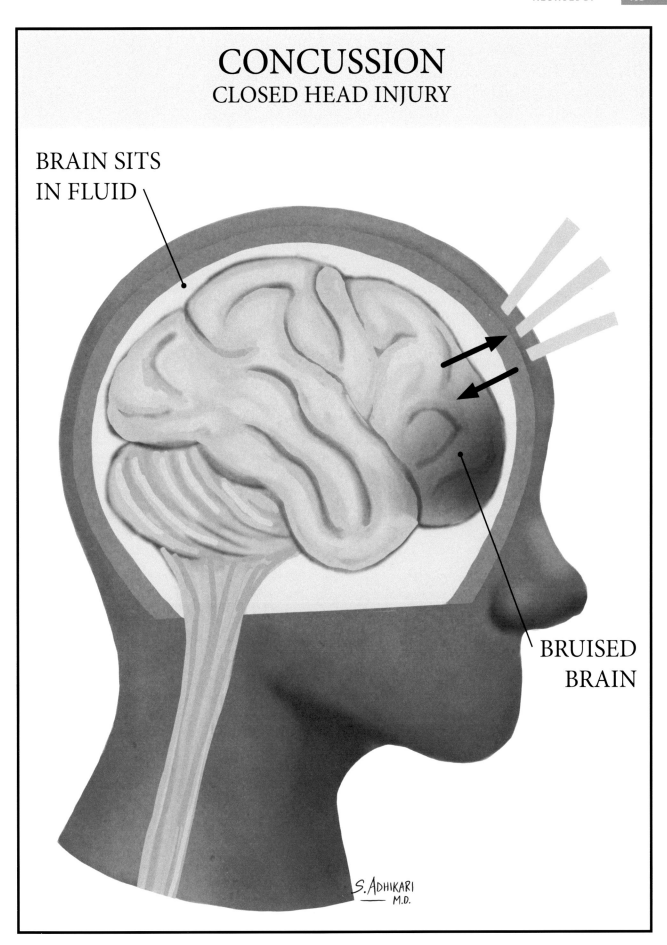

BRUISED
BRAIN

S. ADHIKARI
M.D.

MISCELLANEOUS

CANCER
DIAGNOSIS & WORK-UP

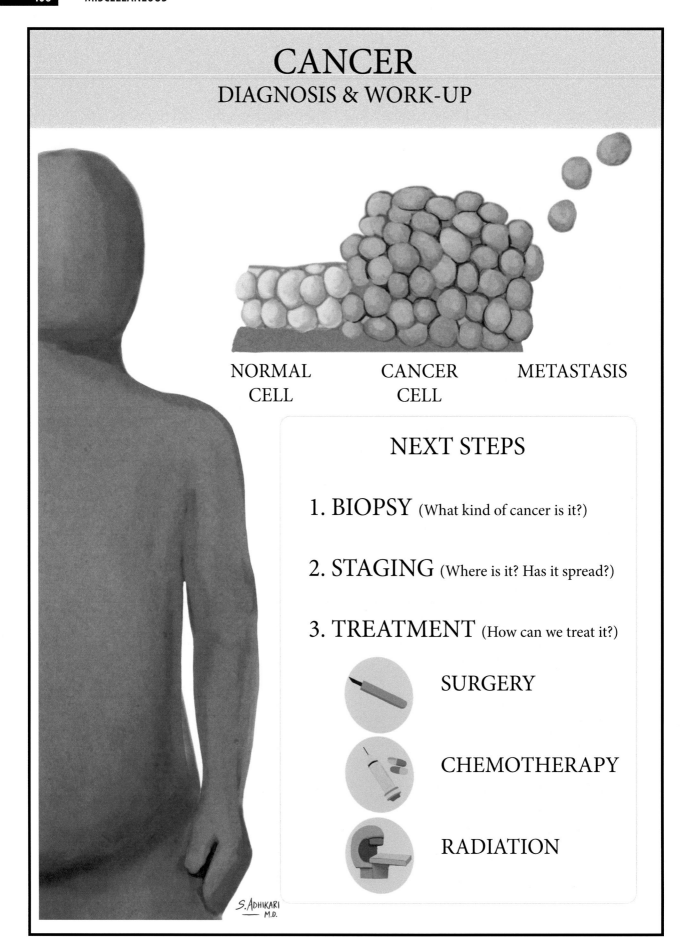

NORMAL   CANCER   METASTASIS
CELL   CELL

NEXT STEPS

1. BIOPSY (What kind of cancer is it?)

2. STAGING (Where is it? Has it spread?)

3. TREATMENT (How can we treat it?)

SURGERY

CHEMOTHERAPY

RADIATION

S. ADHIKARI
M.D.

DIABETES
DIABETES MELLITUS TYPE 2

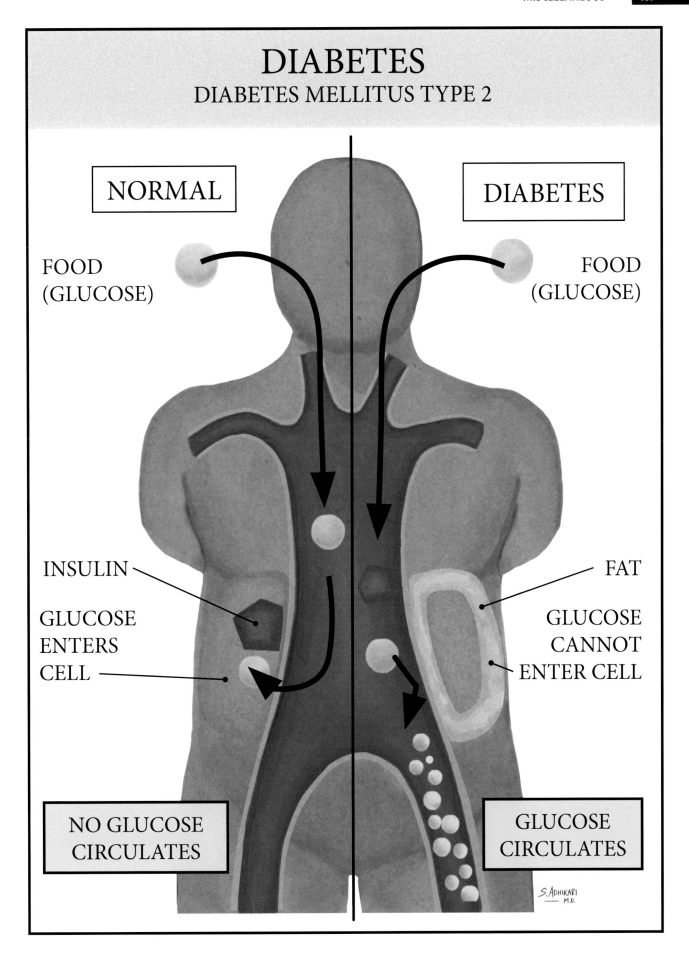

NORMAL

DIABETES

FOOD
(GLUCOSE)

FOOD
(GLUCOSE)

INSULIN

FAT

GLUCOSE
ENTERS
CELL

GLUCOSE
CANNOT
ENTER CELL

NO GLUCOSE
CIRCULATES

GLUCOSE
CIRCULATES

S. ADHIKARI
M.D.

ALTERNATING MEDICATIONS
FEVER CONTROL OR PAIN CONTROL

TIME
(HOUR)

0
1
2
3
4
5
6
7
8
9
10
11
12
....

ACETAMINOPHEN
TYLENOL

IBUPROFEN
MOTRIN, ADVIL

S. ADHIKARI
M.D.

BACTERIA vs VIRUS

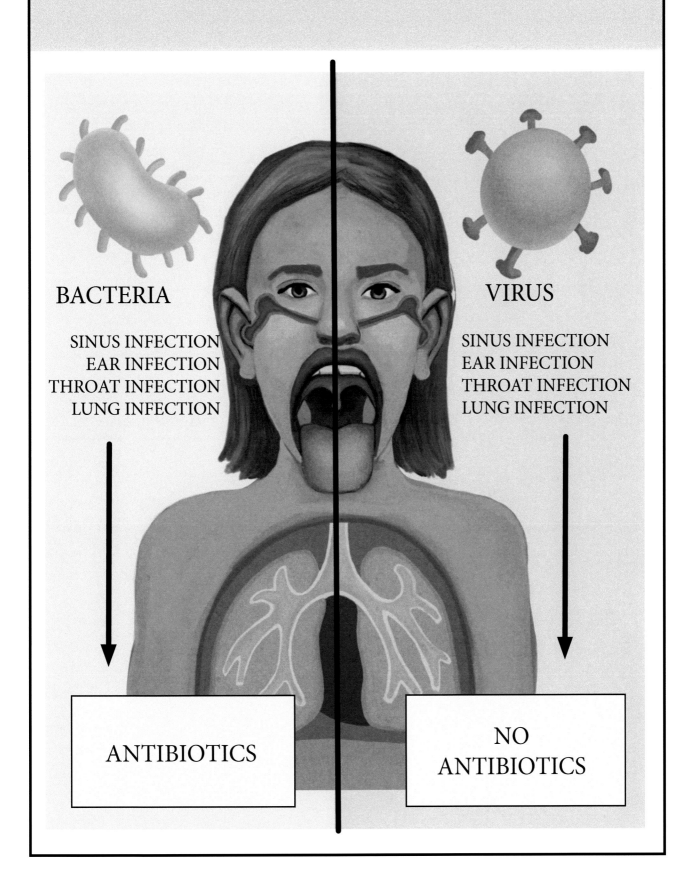

CODE STATUS

FULL CODE

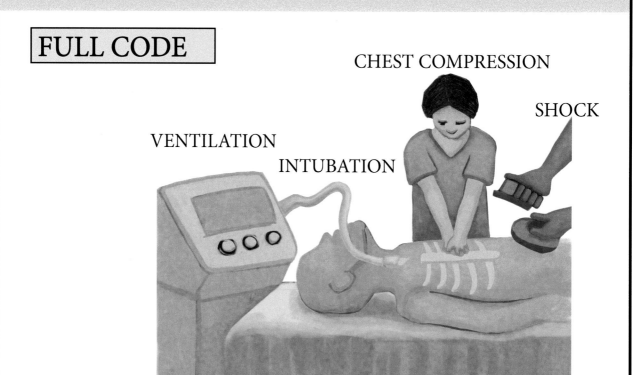

CHEST COMPRESSION

SHOCK

VENTILATION

INTUBATION

DNR/DNI

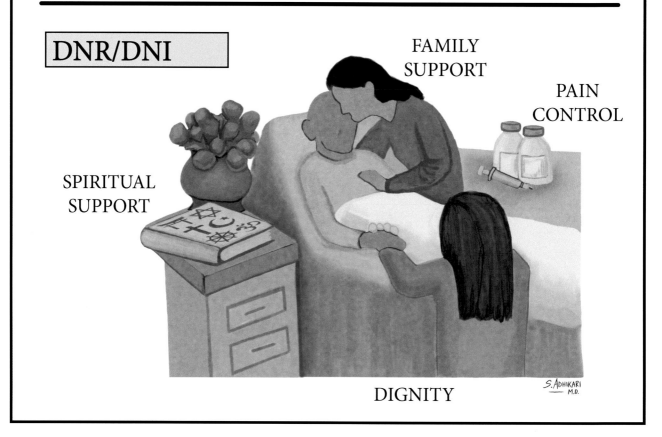

FAMILY SUPPORT

PAIN CONTROL

SPIRITUAL SUPPORT

DIGNITY

SCRIPTING

The images in this book can be used in any way that may be helpful for the patient encounter. A few things are important to keep in mind for effective patient communication:

- Use colloquial terms (e.g.: eardrum instead of tympanic membrane, blood clot instead of pulmonary embolism)
- Focus on the top three things that are pertinent. As clinicians, we know that there may be several differentials that we consider when making diagnoses. However, when talking with a patient, discuss only the most pertinent few.
- Compare the normal ("This is what it is supposed to look like") to the abnormal ("This is what it looks like")
- Address common misconceptions up front
- Discuss the medical lingo and explain what "patients" call it and what "medical professionals" call it.
- Use short sentences that are to the point.

Each patient encounter will be different. The same image may be used multiple times, yet explained in multiple different ways. You may use the same image multiple times, yet explain it in multiple different ways. Some images may be more useful than others. Below are very basic suggestions of how to use a particular image to talk with a patient (each entry corresponds to a page in the book). Notice that each title is written in a colloquial language with the medical terminology listed underneath. Notice also that the labels are also written in a very colloquial language to simplify what is happening for a non-medical patient. Common misconceptions are in *italics*.

SKIN	
Blood draw (Page 2) A tourniquet plumps up your blood vessel (vein). A needle is inserted directly into your vein. Blood is removed. Once the needle is removed, there is no direct access to the blood vessel. To get more blood, a needle needs to be re-inserted. *Clinicians often call this a "butterfly" stick because the device looks like a butterfly.*	**IV (Page 3)** **Intravenous insertion** A tourniquet plumps up your blood vessel (vein). A needle, attached to a small piece of plastic, is inserted directly into your vein. Once inside the vein, the plastic is advanced and the needle is withdrawn. Now, there is direct access to your blood vessels. You can receive fluids or medications through this conduit. A needle does not need to be used again. *The needle does not stay in your blood vessel; only a flexible piece of plastic is left in your arm.*
Cut (Page 4) **Laceration** A cut is a break in the skin. Each cut is unique: where it is, how big and how deep it is, how dirty it is, how close it is to important structures like tendons, blood vessels, and nerves. Some cuts require repair. An abrasion occurs when the skin has rubbed against something and is missing a layer. A puncture wound occurs when there is a deep, narrow break in the skin.	**Options for repair (Page 5)** Repairable lacerations can be fixed using 4 different methods: stitches, Steri-Strips, staples, and adhesive glue. Abrasions usually do not require repair. They slowly fill in over time. *Any time there is a break in the skin, there will be some level of scarring. Clinicians try to minimize any scarring using the appropriate repair technique.*

Boil (Page 6) Abscess Just under our skin, hair follicles contain small glands that secrete sebum. This keeps skin moist and lubricated. When a hair follicle clogs up, the sebum gets trapped under the skin. This forms an early abscess. Sometimes early abscesses resolve on their own. Other times, they need to be cut open with a scalpel.	**MRSA (Page 7)** Methicillin-resistant *Staphylococcus aureus* (MRSA) Our skin is covered with all types of bacteria; MRSA is the name of just one of them. The bottom image depicts how the skin gets infected. The left part of the image depicts normal, intact skin. Here, bacteria on the outside does not enter. The right part of the image depicts broken skin. Here, bacteria enter and infect underlying skin structures. MRSA commonly causes skin ulceration, but can also cause an abscess.
Paronychia (Page 8) Your cuticle sits on top of the nail and helps protect it. Sometimes, bacteria becomes trapped between the cuticle and the nail. A localized infection, called paronychia, develops. To treat a paronychia, simply take a scalpel and lift up the cuticle and drain this collection of pus.	**Crushed finger (Page 9)** Subungual hematoma When you crush the tip of your finger, blood vessels under your nail burst. This causes a lot of pressure and pain. To relieve some of this pressure, a small instrument, called a trephinator, burns a small hole through the nail. Blood drains out, and the pressure is relieved.
Superficial clot (Page 10) Superficial thrombophlebitis Veins return blood to the heart. Our bodies have superficial veins and deeper veins. Sometimes a blood clot develops in these veins. When the clot is in the superficial vein, it causes local inflammation of the wall of the blood vessel. It usually occurs after an IV has been placed. It resolves with heat and time. However, when the clot is in the deep vein, it can be dangerous. It may break off and travel to vital organs, like the lungs.	**Airway anatomy (Page 11)** When you breathe, air flows down past the epiglottis, into your lungs. When you swallow food, the epiglottis acts like a lid and shuts the opening of the airway. This ensures that food goes into the esophagus, instead of the lungs. When you have an allergic reaction or angioedema, the tongue becomes swollen and blocks your airway. When you have epiglottitis, your epiglottis becomes swollen and blocks your airway. When you aspirate, food goes down the wrong tube; it goes down into the lungs instead of the esophagus.
EENT (Eye, ear, nose, throat)	
Eye pain (Page 14) Corneal abrasion & conjunctivitis The surface of the eye is covered with the cornea (over the eye) and the conjunctiva (on the inner surface of the eyelids). The top image depicts the normal side view of the eye. The bottom image depicts a problem with this surface. The left part of the image depicts conjunctivitis. This is where the conjunctiva becomes infected by a virus or a bacteria. The right part of the image depicts a corneal abrasion. This is a scratch on the cornea. A corneal ulcer is a hole through the surface of the cornea.	Toothache (Page 15) Dental caries vs dental abscess The left image depicts a normal tooth. Notice that the nerve sits deep inside the pulp. The right image depicts an abnormal tooth. The left side of the image shows a cracked tooth with an exposed nerve. This causes a lot of pain. The right side of the image shows a cavity that has invaded into the pulp. Bacteria in your mouth travels down into your pulp and forms an abscess.

Nosebleed (Page 16) Epistaxis Many blood vessels lay just under the surface of the nasal mucosa, right next to your nasal septum. Notice how superficial these vessels are. Minor trauma (picking the nose, bumping nose, dry air) can cause a nosebleed. When you have a nose bleed, tilt your head forward and pinch the area just under your bony ridge. If this does not stop the bleeding, you may need nasal packing. A packing puts direct and constant pressure on the area that is bleeding deeper inside the nose. You will go home with this packing. The hole will close up over the next few days. *Do not try to remove the packing by yourself because it may cause more damage.*	**Sinus infection (Page 17)** Sinusitis The sinuses are hollow cavities in your face. The left image depicts a normal sinus. Notice that the sinus drains into your nasal cavity and then out through your nose. The right image depicts sinusitis. Here, the nasal cavities become swollen and block the normal drainage of the sinus. Fluid builds up and accumulates in the sinuses and becomes infected.
Inner ear infection (Page 18) Otitis media The left image depicts normal ear anatomy. Notice the position of the eardrum and the Eustachian tube that connects the ear to the nose. Because of this connection, ear pain is often accompanied by nasal and throat symptoms. The image on the right depicts otitis media or an inner ear infection. Here, fluid accumulates in the area and causes the eardrum to bulge.	**Swimmer's ear (Page 19)** Otitis externa The left image depicts normal ear anatomy. Notice that your ear canal curves around the side of your face. Sometimes, water gets trapped inside and causes an infection. The right image depicts an outer ear infection. Here, the ear canal becomes irritated and pus forms and drains out of the ear.
Sore throat (Page 20) Strep pharyngitis & peritonsillar abscess (PTA) The left image depicts a normal tonsil. It hides between the folds of your throat. The structure that hangs in the middle is called the uvula. The right image depicts an infected tonsil. Notice that the tonsil becomes covered with pus and becomes enlarged and "angry." This is strep throat. Sometimes, the infection spreads beyond the tonsils and into the nearby tissues. Here, it can form into an abscess. This causes the uvula to shift left. When you develop an infection in your throat, your lymph nodes along the side of your neck become swollen as your body fights off the infection.	

CARDIOPULMONARY

Bronchitis vs pneumonia (Page 22)

Both bronchitis and pneumonia present similarly: cough, wheezing, shortness of breath. The left image depicts bronchitis. Notice that there is a problem with the tubes of your airway. They either fill up with mucus, causing a productive cough, OR they spasm and cause wheezing. The right image depicts pneumonia. Notice that there is a problem with your lung tissue itself. Here, the tissue gets infected. Sometimes a chest x-ray can help differentiate the two.

Emphysema (Page 23)
Chronic obstructive pulmonary disease (COPD)

The left image depicts a normal lung. Notice that air moves down the airway. It travels to the alveoli and oxygen gets dropped off, where it then circulates in the bloodstream. Normally, airflow is smooth. The right image depicts a lung with COPD. Notice that the walls of the alveoli are destroyed. Airflow through the airways is not smooth. Instead, muscles that surround the airways spasm and cause bumpy airflow and poor oxygen exchange. Also, airways fill up with mucus and interfere with oxygen exchange.

Blood clot (Page 24)
Deep vein thrombosis (DVT) & pulmonary embolism (PE)

Veins return blood back to your heart and lungs. The left side depicts normal venous return. The right side depicts a blood clot that forms in one of the deep veins of your leg. This causes the leg to swell. Sometimes, a small piece, called an embolism, breaks off and travels to the lungs. When it gets to the lungs, it is called a pulmonary embolism. Here, it blocks oxygen exchange in the lung tissue. The lung tissue dies from the lack of oxygen. This is called a lung infarct.

Swollen legs (Page 25)
Pedal edema

Veins have valves that return blood back to your heart. The left side depicts normal blood return. Notice the valve opens to allow blood to pass and then closes to prevent backflow. This process repeats to bring blood back to the heart. The right image depicts pedal edema. Notice that the valves don't open and close properly. Blood pools at the feet. This extra fluid then seeps into the subcutaneous tissue and causes a "doughy" swelling to the legs.

Heart attack (Page 26)
Myocardial infarction (MI)

The heart is a muscle and needs oxygen just like any other muscle of your body. Coronary arteries supply this oxygen to the heart muscle. Sometimes, the coronary artery gets clogged. When oxygen doesn't reach the muscle, it dies. This is a heart attack.

Chest pain evaluation (Page 27)

When you have chest pain, you may be concerned mainly about your heart. But remember, that your pain may be caused by many other structures that are nearby: the skin, the muscles, the lungs, the stomach, the gallbladder, or the pancreas. Sometimes, we cannot determine the exact cause of your chest pain but have evaluated all of the structures in and around your chest.

Heart failure (Page 28)
Congestive heart failure (CHF)

Think of your heart as a pump: It takes blood in and pumps it out to the rest of your body. Sometimes, your pump fails, and it cannot pump blood out to the rest of the body. Because this incoming blood does not get pumped out, it backs up in your lungs and/or legs.

Heart failure causes (Page 29)
Diastolic vs systolic disease

Heart failure occurs because of two processes. The left image shows diastolic disease. Here, your blood pressure is very high because your blood vessels are very stiff and narrow. Your heart works really hard to pump out blood against this resistance. At first, it keeps up. But, after time, the heart muscle gets really muscular. It has a hard time filling up properly and also a hard time pumping out blood. The right image depicts systolic disease. Here, your heart is weak and dilated (usually because of a heart attack). It just does not have the strength to pump blood out.

High blood pressure (Page 30)
Hypertension (HTN)
The left image depicts normal blood flow out of the heart. Notice that the blood flows smoothly. The right image depicts hypertension. Here, blood flows out of the heart into a stiff, narrow blood vessel. This puts a strain on the heart. The heart muscle enlarges and becomes muscular. You can actually see this on an EKG.
Your blood pressure fluctuates throughout the day (it is usually lowest while sleeping and highest in the evening). It can increase based on emotions (anger, excitement, nervousness). An isolated spike is not concerning if it occurs without symptoms. *It can actually be dangerous to acutely lower your blood pressure if you have no symptoms.* It is the general trend over time (weeks, months) that is very important to prevent the consequences of high blood pressure (kidney failure, stroke, heart attack, etc.).

HTN + symptoms (Page 31)
Hypertensive urgency
So, when should you worry about high blood pressure? When you have symptoms: severe headache/stroke-like symptoms, chest pain, shortness of breath, abdominal pain, back pain, or foot pain. These symptoms tell us that your blood pressure is too high and is causing strain and even damage to the organ.

Irregular heart beat (Page 32)
Atrial fibrillation
The left image depicts the normal electrical impulses that cause the heart to pump in a regular way. Notice the impulse starts in one spot of the heart and then follows in a regular, predictable pathway. This causes a regular, rhythmic beat to the heart. The right image depicts atrial fibrillation. Here, multiple spots fire all at once. This causes a very irregular beating of the heart. During atrial fibrillation, the heart does not empty completely. Clots form in the cavities of the heart. Sometimes, a small piece of this clot breaks off and goes to the brain. Here, it blocks a blood vessel and causes a stroke.

Fluid around heart (Page 33)
Pericarditis vs pericardial effusion
The left image depicts the pericardium, a thin, fibrous structure that surrounds the heart muscle. The right image depicts an inflammation of the pericardium. This is called pericarditis. Sometimes, this inflammation causes fluid to build up in the space between the pericardium and the heart. This fluid is called a pericardial effusion. This can be dangerous because this extra fluid can compress the actual heart muscle and block blood return to the heart.

Aortic dissection (Page 34)
The aorta is a big blood vessel that carries blood from the heart to the rest of the body. It is made up of several layers. Sometimes, the inner wall of the aorta weakens and tears. This is because of high blood pressure. Instead of going down the normal tract, blood enters the wall of the aorta and "bleeds into itself."

Aortic aneurysm (Page 35)
The aorta is a big blood vessel that carries blood from the heart to the rest of the body. Sometimes, the aorta forms a balloon-like bulge. This is called an aneurysm. Sometimes, the pressure gets too high, and the aneurysm ruptures.

Poor circulation (Page 36)
Peripheral artery disease & venous insufficiency
The left image depicts normal circulation. Arteries carry fresh, oxygenated blood to the tissue, and veins return old, deoxygenated blood to the heart. This keeps your tissues healthy. The right image depicts poor circulation. This occurs because of either poor arterial flow or poor venous return. When the artery is involved, it is usually due to clogging of the artery. It can progress to total occlusion and a completely dead toe/foot. When the veins are involved, it is usually due to blood that just sits around in the veins (venous stasis). Poor circulation commonly results in ulcers, or breaks in the skin, that don't heal properly.

GASTROINTESTINAL

Digestion (Page 38)
Think of your digestive system as one long continuous tube. Start at your mouth, down the esophagus, to the stomach, small intestine, large intestine, and then finally the rectum. When food reaches the small intestine, the gallbladder and pancreas (green) send chemicals to help break down the food. Food gets absorbed into the bloodstream and circulates to provide energy to the rest of your body.

Abdominal pain (Page 39)
Sometimes we cannot determine the exact cause of your abdominal pain. We look at all of the organs in the abdomen, as well as the surrounding structures: the heart, the lungs, the bladder, and the reproductive organs. The nerves of the abdomen are visceral, which means they are often vague and not localized. This is different from other nerves of the body that are more localized. This is why it is sometimes difficult to precisely identify the cause of pain.

Heartburn (Page 40)
Gastroesophageal reflux disease (GERD)
Your stomach is full of acid. Normally, this acid stays in your stomach because of a sphincter. This sphincter opens to let food in and closes to keep the acid from going up the esophagus. In GERD, this sphincter relaxes, and stomach acid travels up your esophagus and causes a burning sensation in your chest. It is called "heartburn" because your esophagus sits right behind your heart.

Gastritis & ulcer (Page 41)
Your stomach is full of acid. Usually, protective measures prevent this acid from irritating the wall of the stomach. In gastritis, these protective measures fail and stomach acid eats away at the inner surface of the stomach. If this continues, gastritis can lead to an ulcer, which is an actual hole in the surface of the stomach.

Vomiting blood (Page 42)
Upper gastrointestinal bleed (UGIB)
Your stomach is full of acid. Sometimes, this acid eats away at the surface of the stomach and causes an ulcer. If your ulcer becomes deep enough, it can erode the underlying blood vessel and cause bleeding in the GI tract. Blood can go either up or down. If it goes up (vomit), it looks like coffee grounds. If it goes down (stool), it looks black. *Bleeding in the GI tract can be dangerous because it may be hard to stop the bleeding. When you cut your arm, you can put localized pressure to stop the bleeding. However, when you bleed internally, you cannot put localized pressure to stop the bleeding.*

Rectal bleed (Page 43)
Lower gastrointestinal bleed (LGIB)
When bleeding occurs below the stomach, it is considered a lower gastrointestinal bleed. There are several sources of lower tract bleeding: a polyp, an AVM (an abnormal blood vessel), a diverticular bleed, hemorrhoids. The color of your stool, the briskness of the bleeding, and your medical history can help determine where the bleeding is coming from. Often, we will need to run further tests.

Hiatal hernia (Page 44)

Your esophagus is separated from your stomach by a large muscle called the diaphragm. The esophagus enters through a small hole in the diaphragm. A sphincter opens to let food in and closes to keep acid from going up into the esophagus. Sometimes, the hole in the diaphragm where the esophagus enters grows big. The upper part of the stomach bulges through this hole and enters the chest cavity. This messes up the sphincter so that it cannot open and close properly. Instead, the sphincter just stays open. Stomach acid constantly goes up into the chest and "burns" the esophagus, causing GERD symptoms.

Hernia (Page 45)
Normal vs incarcerated

Hernias occur when there is a weakness in the wall of the abdomen. Sometimes, when you stand up or strain, pressure builds up in your abdominal cavity. Your tissues squeeze out through this weakness. This causes a bulge, or hernia. When you lay down or relax, the hernia usually relaxes and goes back into your abdominal cavity. Sometimes, when your hernia comes out, the tissues swell, and the hernia gets stuck outside your stomach. You cannot push it back inside. Its blood supply gets cut off, and this piece of tissue actually dies.

Foreign body in esophagus (Page 46)
Esophageal stricture

Food normally goes down the esophagus and into the stomach. Sometimes, there is a narrowing of the esophagus, and food gets stuck. This narrowing occurs due to scar tissue, usually due to chronic gastric reflux, a mass, or a nerve problem. When you try to drink water, it comes back up. Sometimes, you may even have a hard time holding your saliva. Sometimes medicines work to relieve this problem; other times, you may need to have an endoscopy to help relieve this obstruction.

Bowel blockage (Page 47)
Small bowel obstruction (SBO)

Think of your digestive system as one long continuous tube. Sometimes, this tube gets blocked and causes a bowel obstruction. Nothing can pass through, and your abdomen gets distended and you may vomit. This blockage can occur due to scar tissue (from previous surgery), a mass, or an internal hernia. To treat this blockage, you need a nasogastric tube (NG tube). This tube is placed through your nose, down your esophagus, and into your stomach. It is hooked up to suction, and everything is sucked out. Sometimes this resolves the blockage because it decompresses the intestines. If it doesn't resolve the blockage, you may need surgery.

Gallbladder disease (Page 48)
Biliary colic

The gallbladder makes chemicals that help digest fatty foods. Sometimes, stones develop in the gallbladder. These stones do not cause much pain when they are in the gallbladder. But, when they start to travel down the bile tracts, they can get stuck. This blocks the gallbladder, and the gallbladder gets infected and its wall thickens. Depending on where the stone gets stuck, it can also cause problems with the liver and the pancreas.

Pancreatitis (Page 49)

The pancreas makes chemicals that help digest foods. Sometimes, the pancreas gets inflamed. This causes upper abdominal pain and vomiting. Many things can cause this inflammation, including alcohol abuse and gallbladder disease. To treat inflamed pancreatitis, you let it rest. Stick to a liquid diet so that you do not stimulate the pancreas to make these chemicals.

Diverticular disease (Page 50)
Diverticulosis, diverticulitis & perforation

On your large intestine, small outpouchings called diverticulosis occur, usually due to chronic constipation or age. In these outpouchings, small particles get stuck and cause inflammation. This is called diverticulitis. If this inflammation becomes severe, the pressure inside causes it to burst (perforate), and the contents of your gut spill out into the abdominal cavity.

Constipation (Page 51)

Constipation occurs when your stool gets backed up in your colon. This backup can occur over several days to weeks. *There is no quick fix for this problem.* Enemas help lubricate the stool in the lower part of the colon, but they only extend so far. Oral medications, like stool softeners, work if the stool is higher up but may take 1–2 days to become effective.

Perirectal abscess (Page 52) There are muscles that control the opening and closing of your rectum. Sometimes, you may develop an abscess in this area. If superficial, we can drain them. If they are deeper, they may require an operation.	**Hemorrhoids (Page 53)** Hemorrhoids are enlarged blood vessels that are close to the rectum. They can be internal or external. Sometimes, they bleed when hard pieces of stool rub up against and nick them. Usually, the blood will be bright red.
Appendicitis (Page 54) The appendix is located in your right lower abdomen and is attached to your intestine. Sometimes, a small piece of stool, called a fecalith, gets stuck at the opening of the appendix. The appendix gets swollen, and you develop appendicitis.	

GENITOURINARY

Kidney stone (Page 56) **Nephrolithiasis** The kidney is connected to the bladder with a small tube called the ureter. Kidney stones form in the kidney. Usually, they do not cause pain here because there is a lot of space to move around. As kidney stones travel down the ureter, they cause a "colicky" type of pain that comes and goes. Sometimes, these stones become stuck at the junction between the ureter and the bladder. When this happens, the area behind the obstructed stone dilates. Stones that are less than 5 mm usually pass on their own. Stones that are larger than 5 mm may require intervention to pass.	**Urinary tract infection (Page 57)** **Cystitis vs pyelonephritis** The urinary tract consists of several structures: the urethra, the bladder, the ureters, and the kidneys. Infections can occur anywhere along the tract. Bladder infections, when left untreated, can progress to a kidney infection.
Enlarged prostate (Page 58) **Benign prostatic hypertrophy (BPH)** The prostate gland sits just under the bladder. As we age, it grows bigger and blocks the bladder, making it difficult to pass urine. In the beginning, urine flows in a weak stream. With time, urine flow becomes completely blocked. When the prostate blocks urine flow, urine sits around in the bladder and becomes infected. Sometimes, it travels up to the kidneys and causes a kidney infection.	**Urinary retention (Page 59)** When the prostate gland completely blocks the bladder, you cannot urinate. Your bladder distends and you feel pain. A foley catheter is placed to relieve this blockage. This stiff piece of plastic enters the urethra and pushes the prostate gland to the side. It makes a track so that urine can flow again. The foley catheter stays for a few days. *Do not pull out your catheter; notice there is a balloon at the end that keeps it in place. If you try to pull it out without deflating the balloon first, it will damage your organs.*
Testicular swelling (Page 60) **Epididymitis** The epididymis is a curved structure just above the testicles. Sometimes, it gets infected. This causes pain and swelling to the testicle. It is often treated with antibiotics.	**Testicular swelling (Page 61)** **Hydrocele vs. varicocele** Hydrocele occurs when a sac of fluid collects in the testicle. It causes testicular swelling and pain. It can develop with trauma or inflammation. It usually goes away with time. Varicocele is when the blood vessels to the testicles engorge. This causes pain and swelling. This is similar to the varicose veins you may see in your legs.

Testicular torsion (Page 62) Sometimes, the testicle twists around and around. Its blood supply gets cut off. The testicle dies. This causes severe pain. This is an emergency.	**Ovarian torsion (Page 63)** Sometimes, the ovary twists around and around. Its blood supply gets cut off. The ovary dies. This causes severe pain. This is an emergency.
Ovarian cyst (Page 64) Normal cyst vs ruptured cyst Every month, your ovary produces an egg. This egg travels to the uterus and waits to get fertilized. This is called ovulation. During this process, a cyst can also develop on the surface of the ovary. The cysts fill with either fluid or blood. When they rupture, the fluid collects in the abdominal cavity and causes pain. Blood is especially irritating to the abdominal cavity. *This fluid does not connect to the outside world (you will not expel it during menstruation); instead, the fluid gets resorbed into our bodies over several days.*	**Early pregnancy (Page 65)** Abdominal pain &/or vaginal bleeding During early pregnancy, sometimes an ultrasound is inconclusive. We cannot actually see the baby inside the uterus, where it is supposed to be. When this happens, there could be three possibilities. First, it is just too early, and everything is just too small. Second, you are having a miscarriage, and the baby is on its way out. Third, the baby is in the tubes (instead of the uterus). This is called an ectopic pregnancy. It can be quite dangerous because the tube can rupture and cause lots of bleeding. Time will tell which one of these possibilities you have. This is why it is very important to follow up in 2 days to get more blood work.
Fibroids (Page 66) Leiomyoma Fibroids are non-cancerous growths on the wall of the uterus. They can grow anywhere in the uterus. Sometimes they cause heavy vaginal bleeding. This happens especially when they sit just under the surface of the uterus wall. They get bigger with hormones; they shrink during menopause.	**Irregular periods (Page 67)** Abnormal uterine bleeding Every month, blood builds up in the uterus. This happens because of hormones. Normally, these hormones cycle in a regular fashion; you have regular periods that come once a month. Sometimes, the hormones cycle in an irregular fashion; this causes irregular periods. The periods can be heavier than usual, more painful than usual, or come at irregular intervals. Lots of things affect the cyclical pattern of hormones: stress, low or high body weight, medicines, or hormonal imbalances.
Yeast infection (Page 68) Vaginal candidiasis Fungus likes moist, warm, dark places like the vagina. It can grow and cause a lot of irritation and itchiness and a lot of cottage cheese–like discharge.	**Vaginal discharge (Page 69)** Bacterial vaginosis Normally, there is a delicate balance between "good" bacteria and "bad" bacteria in the vagina. This balance keeps everything stable. Sometimes, there is an overgrowth of the bad bacteria in the vagina. This is called bacterial vaginosis. People usually present with vaginal discharge and odor.
Pelvic infection (Page 70) Pelvic inflammatory disease (PID) & tubo-ovarian abscess (TOA) Sometimes, you can get an infection in the uterus. This is commonly caused by a sexually transmitted infection. STIs first infect the vagina and then proceed upward into the uterus. It then causes an infection. This is called pelvic inflammatory disease. Sometimes the infection can travel even further into the tubes and cause an abscess.	**Sexually transmitted infection (Page 71)** Infections that are transmitted through sexual contact are called sexually transmitted infections. Common infections are gonorrhea, chlamydia, trichomonas, herpes, syphilis, and HIV. Many times, these infections present with symptoms like discharge, itchiness, or odor. However, other times, the infection can have no symptoms. *STIs can occur anywhere there is sexual contact (genitals, mouth, anus, skin).*

Lower abdomen (Page 72) **Male vs female** Male and females have distinct anatomy. Males have two exits: the rectum (stool) and the urethra (urine). Females have three exits: the rectum (stool), the vagina, and the urethra (urine). The male's exits are further apart, anatomically than the female's exits. This makes urinary tract infections much more common in females than in males. Why? Bacteria from the rectum (GI tract) travels to the bladder, causing a urinary tract infection.	

ORTHOPEDICS

Broken (Page 74) **Fracture** A broken bone is the same thing as a fractured bone. There are many different types of fractures. Different types of fractures require different treatments.	**Growth plate injury (Page 75)** Growth plates are areas at the ends of your long bones where new bone growth occurs. The left image shows the location of the growth plate. The middle image depicts how the growth plate adds new bone to existing bone. This allows the bone to grow longer. The right image depicts an injury to the growth plate. Here, new bone growth is disrupted. The bone does not form normally. Injuries to the growth plate are especially important to take care of properly.
Arthritis (Page 76) **Degenerative joint disease** There are many different types of arthritis. The most common type is called osteoarthritis and occurs due to the aging process; essentially, it is "wear-and-tear" arthritis. The left images depict normal joints (top is a hip joint; bottom is the spine). Notice that the bones are smooth and regular. The right image depicts arthritic joints. Notice that the bones are ratty and irregular. Normal joints are covered with spongy cartilage that helps protect them. Arthritic joints have worn-down cartilage and exposed bone. Arthritic joints result in bone hitting against other bones, causing inflammation and pain. It can also cause the growth of bony spurs (osteophytes). Arthritis occurs over many years and is irreversible.	**Bursitis (Page 77)** A bursa is a fluid-filled sac. It sits right between your muscle and your bone. The bursa helps to protect against constant rubbing. This is especially important at your larger joints, which are constantly moving (i.e. hip, shoulder, knee). Sometimes, with repeated activity, your bursa becomes inflamed. This results in pain and swelling.

Rib fracture (Page 78) The rib cage is an interconnected group of several bones. When you break just one rib, you can have a lot of pain because this one rib belongs to an entire structure. This differs from breaking your arm. With a broken arm, you can isolate just that bone and immobilize it with a cast. If you break a rib, you cannot isolate or immobilize it. Every time you breathe, you irritate the fracture. You tend to take shallow breaths and don't expand your entire lungs. This sets you up for pneumonia. *Rib fractures do not always show up on chest x-rays because there are so many overlapping structures.*	**Collapsed lung (Page 79)** Pneumothorax The left side of the image depicts your normal lung anatomy. Notice that your lungs are covered with a small layer of tissue that is continuous with a small layer that sits just underneath the rib cage. The right side of the image depicts a collapsed lung. Here, air leaks into the space between these two layers. It builds up and eventually causes the lung to collapse. When your lung collapses, you need a chest tube, which removes the air trapped in this space.
Back pain (Page 80) Musculoskeletal Our bodies are covered with muscles. A very common cause of back pain is muscular strain. Strained muscles usually feel sore and achy several hours to several days after exertion or activity.	**Back pain (Page 81)** Sacroiliitis Sacroiliitis is a common cause of back pain. Sacroiliitis occurs because there is inflammation at the joint between the spine and the pelvis. Usually, you have pain in the lower back, in the buttocks, and down the back of your legs. It gets worse after standing or sitting for long periods of time.
Back pain (Page 82) Side view There are many different causes of lower back pain. The left image depicts a side view of the back. The right image depicts the different structures. From the outside, there is a layer of muscle. It is common for these muscles to get strained. Going deeper, there is the column of bones that surround the spinal cord. And finally, there is the spinal cord with several nerve roots coming out of it. As you can see, finding the exact cause of back pain can be difficult as there are so many structures involved.	**Sciatica (Page 83)** Lumbar radiculopathy The sciatic nerve exits the spinal cord near the buttocks and runs down the back of your leg. Sometimes, the sciatic nerve gets irritated. The image on your right depicts how the sciatic nerve gets damaged. Notice that the nerve can get compressed by a bulging disk, a bony fragment, or a muscle spasm.
Neck pain (Page 84) Cervical strain There are several different causes of neck pain. The left image depicts a side view of the neck. The right image depicts the different structures. From the outside, there is a layer of muscle. It is common for these muscles to get strained. Going deeper, there is the column of bones that surround the spinal cord. And finally, there is the spinal cord with several nerve roots coming out of it. As you can see, finding the exact cause of neck pain can be difficult as there are so many structures involved.	**Neck & back strain (Page 85)** Motor vehicle accident (MVA) When you are in a car accident, the muscles all over your body tense up. Often, the large muscles of your neck and lower back get strained. Sometimes the pain starts immediately. However, more commonly the pain begins 6–8 hours after muscle strain. It is similar to going to the gym: You are usually not sore the day you work out, but instead are sore the next few days. *X-rays are helpful when you suspect a broken bone. They are not helpful when you suspect a muscle strain.*

Knee arthritis (Page 86) **Osteoarthritis** Osteoarthritis is often called "wear-and-tear" arthritis because it occurs as we age. The left side depicts a normal knee joint. Notice that there is a layer of cartilage that covers the ends of the bones. This protects the bone. There is also fluid between the bones that help buffer impact. The right side depicts a knee with arthritis. Notice that the cartilage has broken down, and the bones are hitting directly against bone. This causes local inflammation, pain, and degeneration of the bone. Also, the fluid becomes in the joint. *Arthritis is a progressive problem and unfortunately cannot be reversed.*	**Knee pain (Page 87)** **Fracture vs sprain** Often when we injure our knees, we are surprised to find that there is no broken bone (*the x-ray is normal*). This is because there are so many structures in the knee. The left side depicts a normal knee. Notice that in addition to the bones, there are several ligaments that connect the bones together. This helps with the stability of the joint. The far left image shows all of the structures of the knee: the muscles, the patella, the tendon, and the ligament. The right side depicts a sprained knee. Here, the ligaments get partially stretched and even torn. This causes extra fluid to accumulate in the joint. This is called a joint effusion.
Joint disease (Page 88) **Normal anatomy** Every joint in our body is made up of three basic structures: the bone, the cartilage, and the fluid. The fluid helps cushion the ends of the bone and serves as a buffer for impact.	**Inflamed joint (Page 89)** **Gout vs septic joint** The fluid in every joint in your body is called synovial fluid. Sometimes, it gets inflamed or infected. When this happens, you develop a lot of pain every time you move your joint. The left image depicts a joint with gout. Here, crystals form in the fluid. The entire joint becomes inflamed and becomes quite painful to move. The right image depicts a joint that is infected. We call this a "septic joint." Here, the synovial fluid gets infected.
Baker's cyst (Page 90) The fluid between the ends of your bones is called synovial fluid. It helps to cushion your joints against impact. The left image depicts the side view of a normal knee. The right image depicts a knee with a Baker's cyst. Here, the synovial fluid seeps out into the area just behind the knee. You may notice a bulge in this area that may be painful.	**Ankle pain (Page 91)** **Fracture vs sprain** The ankle joint is made up of the bones and the ligaments that hold them together. The left image depicts a broken ankle. You can see this on an x-ray. The right image depicts a sprained ankle. Here, the ligaments get stretched or torn. *You cannot see this on an x-ray.*
Wrist pain (Page 92) **Carpal tunnel syndrome** The carpal tunnel is a small tunnel at your wrist. Nerves and tendons pass underneath this tunnel. With repeated bending back and forth of your wrist, the tendons become inflamed. This puts pressure on the nerve, causing pain, numbness, and tingling in the first three fingers.	**Foot pain (Page 93)** **Plantar fasciitis** There is a thick band of tissue that connects your heel to your toes. Sometimes, this band becomes inflamed, and you develop foot pain.

Broken back (Page 94)
Compression fracture
Our spines are made up of several vertebrae, stacked one on top of another. Each vertebra is named based on where it is located. There are 7 cervical vertebrae, 12 thoracic vertebrae, and 5 lumbar vertebrae. A compression fracture is a fracture to one of these vertebrae.

NEUROLOGY

Stroke (Page 96)
Cerebral vascular accident (CVA)
A stroke occurs when your brain tissue does not get enough oxygen and dies. There are two main types of strokes. The left side depicts a hemorrhagic stroke. Hemorrhage means bleeding. One of the blood vessels in the brain bursts and bleeds into the brain. The brain tissue surrounding this bleeding does not get enough oxygen and dies. This usually happens when your blood pressure is too high. The right side depicts an ischemic stroke. This occurs when your arteries become clogged, which causes decreased blood flow to your brain tissue. Each stroke is different clinically in how it affects you; it depends on what part of your brain is damaged.

Mini-stroke (Page 97)
Transient ischemic attack (TIA)
A ministroke is when you have decreased blood flow to your brain. The brain tissue does not die completely; it just temporarily has decreased blood flow. The left side depicts normal blood flow. Notice all parts of the brain are happy and healthy because they are getting plenty of oxygen. The right side depicts a clogged blood vessel, resulting in temporary decreased blood flow to the brain. Usually, the symptoms resolve once the blood returns. A ministroke is a warning sign. It tells you that a real stroke may soon occur.

Brain bleed (Page 98)
Intracranial hemorrhage (ICH)
The skull is a strong bone that protects the brain. It cannot expand. If you develop bleeding inside your skull, the blood pools inside with nowhere to go. This excess blood puts pressure on your brain tissue and dies. It also squeezes nearby tissue and causes damage. We often talk about the midline shift. This is when the brain pushes across the halfway point; this predicts a very poor prognosis. Brain bleeds can happen either when you just hit your head or when you hit your head and actually break your skull.

Brain aneurysm (Page 99)
Subarachnoid hemorrhage (SAH)
Normally, blood flows to the brain tissue through several different arteries. Sometimes, an artery develops a bulge; this is called an aneurysm. An aneurysm can burst and bleed into the brain. The brain tissue surrounding the blood does not get enough oxygen and dies.

Meningitis (Page 100)
The brain and spinal cord sit in a sac of fluid. Sometimes, this fluid gets infected. You may develop a fever, headache, and neck pain. To determine whether this fluid is infected, we need to perform a lumbar puncture/spinal tap to analyze the fluid.

Dizziness (Page 101)
Benign positional vertigo (BPV)
Semicircular canals are structures that sit deep within the bones behind your ear canal. Fluid fills these canals and moves smoothly as you turn your head left and right. This smooth movement sends signals to the brain through nerves and helps you keep balance. Sometimes, part of the surface of these canals flake off into the fluid. This disrupts the normal flow, and when this happens, you will feel off balance. Dizziness may last anywhere from a few days to several weeks as your body naturally resorbs these flakes.

Bell's palsy (Page 102)
7th cranial nerve palsy
The facial nerve controls the muscles of your face. It is considered a peripheral nerve because it is on the outside of your brain/skull. Sometimes, this nerve gets paralyzed. When this happens, you will not be able to scrunch your forehead, blink your eyes, smile, or taste foods properly. Although this can resemble a stroke, it is not a stroke. Bell's palsy usually lasts for a few days and goes away on its own.

Concussion (Page 103)
Closed head injury
The brain sits in a sac of fluid, which helps protect it from injury. Sometimes, when you hit your head against something hard, the impact moves your brain forward, and it bumps against the inside of your skull. This impact causes a small bruise on the brain tissue itself. The symptoms of a concussion include headache, memory loss, nausea, and confusion.

MISCELLANEOUS

Cancer (Page 106)
Diagnosis & workup
Cancer occurs when a cell in your body grows uncontrollably. The top image depicts normal cell growth. Notice that this cell knows when to stop growing. A cancer cell does not know when to stop growing. Metastasis is when a cancer cell breaks off, travels to another part of the body, and starts to grow there.
Once you find cancer in your body, you need a biopsy. Here, a sample of the cancer is examined under a microscope. Then, you need staging. Here, you need to find out where it is and if it has spread. Usually, this is done with imaging, like a CT scan. Finally, you come up with a treatment plan. You may need (1) surgery to remove cancer, (2) chemotherapy (medicines that kill off cancer), or (3) radiation therapy (radiation to kill cancer cells). You may need a combination of these different types of treatment.

Diabetes (Page 107)
Diabetes mellitus type 2
Diabetes occurs when your body cannot process glucose. The left image depicts your body taking in food (glucose). Normally, your body absorbs the glucose into your cell and uses it for fuel. In diabetes, your cell cannot absorb the glucose, so it circulates in your bloodstream. The inset depicts this process in more detail. Note that insulin, which is made by the pancreas, helps glucose enter the cell. The left side of the image depicts glucose entering the cell normally. Notice that insulin helps glucose enter the cell. The right side of the image depicts diabetes. Here, glucose cannot enter the cell because the cell is covered with fat (adipose), making it "insulin resistant." Because it cannot enter the cell, it continues to circulate in the bloodstream.

Alternating medications (Page 108)
Fever control or pain control
Sometimes, it is necessary to take two different medicines for maximal pain relief or fever control. It is helpful to alternate medications. At "Time Zero," take acetaminophen. Then, 3 hours later, take ibuprofen. Three hours later, take acetaminophen again. It will have been 6 hours since your last dose of acetaminophen. Three hours later, take ibuprofen again. If you stagger your medications, you can safely treat your pain/fever effectively.

Bacteria vs virus (Page 109)
Bacteria and viruses are tiny particles that infect us. They look different and act different, yet they cause similar diseases, especially in the respiratory tract (i.e. sinus, ear, throat, lung). The left image shows a bacteria, and the right image shows a virus. Notice that both can cause a sinus infection, an ear infection, a throat infection, or a lung infection. *The main difference is that bacterial infections are treated with antibiotics; in viral infections, antibiotics do not work.*

Code status (Page 110)
Sometimes, it is necessary to decide what to do if your heart were to stop or if you stopped breathing. Many of the terms medical professionals use can be quite confusing. It is helpful to clarify what types of resuscitation you/your family member would want in this situation. The top image depicts what we call "full code." Here, notice the breathing tube that is placed in your lungs (intubation) and the machine it is hooked to (ventilator). If your heart were to stop, chest compressions would be performed, and if indicated, your body would get electrically shocked. The bottom image depicts what we call "DNR/DNI" (do not resuscitate/do not intubate). Here, notice that you will be kept comfortable with pain medicines or oxygen, be surrounded by family members, have spiritual support, and most of all have dignity in your last moments. *DNR/DNI does not mean do not treat.*

Index

For the benefit of digital users, indexed terms that span two pages (e.g., 52–53) may, on occasion, appear on only one of those pages.